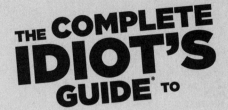

Making Natural Beauty Products

by Sally W. Trew with Zonella B. Gould

ALPHA

A member of Penguin Group (USA) Inc.

ALPHA BOOKS

Published by the Penguin Group

Penguin Group (USA) Inc., 375 Hudson Street, New York, New York 10014, USA

Penguin Group (Canada), 90 Eglinton Avenue East, Suite 700, Toronto, Ontario M4P 2Y3, Canada (a division of Pearson Penguin Canada Inc.)

Penguin Books Ltd., 80 Strand, London WC2R 0RL, England

Penguin Ireland, 25 St. Stephen's Green, Dublin 2, Ireland (a division of Penguin Books Ltd.)

Penguin Group (Australia), 250 Camberwell Road, Camberwell, Victoria 3124, Australia (a division of Pearson Australia Group Pty. Ltd.)

Penguin Books India Pvt. Ltd., 11 Community Centre, Panchsheel Park, New Delhi—110 017, India

Penguin Group (NZ), 67 Apollo Drive, Rosedale, North Shore, Auckland 1311, New Zealand (a division of Pearson New Zealand Ltd.)

Penguin Books (South Africa) (Pty.) Ltd., 24 Sturdee Avenue, Rosebank, Johannesburg 2196, South Africa

Penguin Books Ltd., Registered Offices: 80 Strand, London WC2R 0RL, England

International Standard Book Number: 978-1-61564-023-2
Library of Congress Catalog Card Number: 2010920428

12 11 10   8 7 6 5 4 3 2 1

Interpretation of the printing code: The rightmost number of the first series of numbers is the year of the book's printing; the rightmost number of the second series of numbers is the number of the book's printing. For example, a printing code of 10-1 shows that the first printing occurred in 2010.

Printed in the United States of America

Note: This publication contains the opinions and ideas of its authors. It is intended to provide helpful and informative material on the subject matter covered. It is sold with the understanding that the authors and publisher are not engaged in rendering professional services in the book. If the reader requires personal assistance or advice, a competent professional should be consulted.

The authors and publisher specifically disclaim any responsibility for any liability, loss, or risk, personal or otherwise, which is incurred as a consequence, directly or indirectly, of the use and application of any of the contents of this book.

Most Alpha books are available at special quantity discounts for bulk purchases for sales promotions, premiums, fund-raising, or educational use. Special books, or book excerpts can also be created to fit specific needs.

For details, write: Special Markets, Alpha Books, 375 Hudson Street, New York, NY 10014.

Publisher: *Marie Butler-Knight*
Associate Publisher: *Mike Sanders*
Senior Managing Editor: *Billy Fields*
Acquisitions Editors: *Karyn Gerhard, Tom Stevens*
Senior Development Editor: *Christy Wagner*
Production Editor: *Kayla Dugger*

Copy Editor: *Emily Bell Garner*
Cover Designer: *Kurt Owens*
Book Designers: *William Thomas, Rebecca Batchelor*
Indexer: *Celia McCoy*
Layout: *Brian Massey*
Proofreader: *John Etchison*

Zonella and I both would like to say a special thank you to Ken Bower for creating SoapCalc.
I would like to dedicate my part of this book to my family for all their support and help. —Sally Trew
I would like to dedicate my part of this book to my family for all their support and help. —Zonella Gould

Contents

Appendixes

Introduction

In the early 1970s, I went to beauty school to become a hairdresser. I quickly sped through all the basic classroom work and was soon out on the floor doing hair. It was there that I met an incredible instructor named Marc London. Marc was a very forward-thinking man and had been working with chemists to create his own line of cosmetics. Marc taught me everything he knew about makeup. He and I became close friends, and soon I was helping sell his cosmetics. What did Marc use for his powdered eye shadows? Micas.

I learned so much from Marc, and we remained close friends right up to his death in early 2000. His techniques are the base for all my cosmetic blends and formulations in this book. With my background in art and his teaching, I've been able to create blends and color grinds for all types of mineral makeup products and now share that knowledge with you.

I love to formulate. Give me a challenge, and I will happily meet it. Tell me there's no way to make a product without chemical ingredients, and I won't give up until I've figured out how to make that very product with all-natural ingredients. For this book, that challenge was natural, no-chemical mascara. I have to admit, I almost threw in the towel on that one! Just when I was ready to give up, the last formulation I created worked! Challenge met successfully!

Learning how to make your own beauty products will save you lots of money over the coming years, and that's an important point. However, knowing exactly what ingredients are used and how they work is far more important than the money you'll save. Nature always provides, and we believe natural is best. When using commercial products, you could be using ingredients you don't even know are there. The Food and Drug Administration (FDA) only requires that ingredients used in quantities greater than 1 percent be listed on a product's label. A commercial product may claim to have shea butter, for example, but read the label. You may not find it listed because the manufacturer used less than 1 percent in the formulation.

Think about that for a moment, and you'll realize that the same is true for other ingredients. You might not know everything that's in the product you're buying and using on your skin. When making your own cosmetics, you'll know and control how much of each ingredient you use in your product. That knowledge is worth a million. Who wants to goop chemically made products on their eyes? Wouldn't you prefer to use natural mascara? Some of these natural products might be a little tricky to make at first, but the benefits are worth the trouble when you know you're not using anything that could harm you.

In the chapters about the oils, herbs, and essential oils, you learn so many natural ways to help improve your daily life. We tell you how to use herbs and essential oils to clean the air you breathe in your home, which essential oils can be used on cuts and abrasions, and many more helpful tips.

The co-author relationship Zonella and I have works well because Zonella is the strongest in the areas I'm weakest and vice versa. So we each penned the chapters that highlight our strengths. I have enjoyed formulating and testing the recipes in this book. We hope that you will gain the knowledge from this book to help you live a healthier and greener lifestyle.

So speaking of recipes—and this book contains over 250 of them!—where should you start? I suggest you sample the simple recipes if this is the first time you've attempted to make beauty products. This will be a lot like cooking—there are certain steps when adding dry ingredients to wet, and you may mix two or three things together in one bowl and later add that bowl to a bigger mixture. If you can follow a recipe for cooking, you can follow these recipes, too, and soon will be making your very own natural products. You're going to love this! Try making one of the lotion recipes from Chapter 3. Lotion sounds hard but is actually so easy and fun to make!

How to Use This Book

In this book you learn how to make just about every beauty product you can think of—and make them with all-natural ingredients. Here's how we break it all down:

In **Part 1, Natural Beauty Product Basics,** you learn how to get started—especially how to prepare and sterilize your workplace, equipment, and containers. You also learn all about oils, butters, and herbs, and how to incorporate them into natural beauty products.

In **Part 2, Pampering Skin and Body Products,** we jump right in with facial and clay masks, lotions, creams, body butters, bath bombs, and more. No matter your skin type, you'll find a recipe to use.

In **Part 3, Creating Mineral Makeup,** we give you all the recipes for making foundations, concealers, correctors, blushes, bronzers, eye shadows, lipsticks, lip liners, eyeliners, and mascara. With more than 80 color grinds, you're sure to find the right color for you. We also give you instructions on how to blend colors for your skin type and tone.

We've even dedicated a chapter to the guys—because they need beauty products, too!—with recipes for everything from shaving needs to moisturizers and colognes.

That's the first chapter in **Part 4, For the Fellas and Beyond.** Finally, we close the book with a final chapter of miscellaneous recipes for fun and useful products we couldn't fit in the other chapters.

In the back of the book, you'll find several helpful appendixes, from a glossary; to INCI and FDA labeling guidelines; to a list of resources of our well-known, trusted, and loved suppliers. This book will keep you busy making and enjoying products for years to come!

Extra Bits

Throughout the book, you'll see nuggets of extra information, neatly packaged in sidebar boxes. Here's what to look for:

BEAUTY BIT

These sidebars contain definitions of beauty product–related words you might not yet be familiar with.

IN THE MIRROR

Look to these sidebars for fun and interesting bits of information.

PRETTY POINTER

Be sure to check out these sidebars. They contain helpful hints and tips to make the job easier.

SAFETY FIRST

You'll definitely want to heed the warnings in these sidebars.

Acknowledgments

We would like to say thank you to Jen at Lotion Crafters and Kaila at TKB Trading for all their help and for taking the time out of their busy days to answer questions. It's always a pleasure to talk with you, and you both are always so helpful and willing to share your experience and knowledge. Thank you!

A big shout-out to all the list members of the ApplesNBerries Yahoo! group!

We would also like to thank three great women, Marilyn Allen, Karyn Gerhard, and Christy Wagner. You all worked very hard to make this book a reality.

—Sally Trew

I would like to thank all the people who have given me encouragement to persevere.

—Zonella Gould

Trademarks

All terms mentioned in this book that are known to be or are suspected of being trademarks or service marks have been appropriately capitalized. Alpha Books and Penguin Group (USA) Inc. cannot attest to the accuracy of this information. Use of a term in this book should not be regarded as affecting the validity of any trademark or service mark.

Natural Beauty Product Basics

Welcome to the world of making natural beauty products! Part 1 starts you off at the beginning, explaining why it's better for you to "go natural," and might open your eyes to some of the undesirables used in the commercial beauty products you have been using.

Then we cover everything you need to know about oils and butters used to make natural beauty products, along with yummy essential oils and versatile herbs. This part will become a well-read and -used reference for you when you start to venture into formulating your own recipes and products—and trust us, you will.

The following chapters explain all about the oils and butters and the basic properties and uses for each, so you can better decide what you want in your recipe. Next we look at essential oils. They're so much more than pretty scents! Then we walk through the herb garden. You'll be amazed what these herbs can do besides making your food taste good, especially after you learn how to make infusions and tinctures.

Why Make Your Own?

In This Chapter

- Greening your beauty products
- Tips for keeping your workspace spotless
- The importance of sanitizing your equipment
- What your skin *really* needs to be healthy

Why make your own natural beauty products? A better question might be why *not* make them! There are so many benefits: you get to control what ingredients are and, perhaps more importantly, are *not* used (you can't do that with commercial products); you can create all the colors and scents you love; and by avoiding nasty chemicals, you help protect the earth a little—and each little bit helps!

This book was such a joy to write. We can't wait for you to dig in to all our favorite recipes and start making your own natural beauty products—everything from simple cleansers to mascara. With the recipes in this book, you can be more beautiful and beautifully green, too.

Protect Your Body—and the Earth

Going green. Getting back to basics. These phrases are bandied about a lot these days. But when was the last time you knew where and how your food was grown? Or recognized every ingredient on a food label? Take a look at your cosmetics. Do you recognize all those ingredients, or are most chemicals you've never seen before, let alone recognize? Our lives have become very convenient—and that's not always a bad thing! But when we don't pay attention to the chemicals we use in and on our bodies, and therefore in and on our earth, it might be time to step back and reexamine things a bit.

In the United States, cosmetics don't have to be pretested or approved before they're marketed. That's a shocking but true fact. Reading labels and knowing which chemicals are harmful can make a difference in your life and that of your family's.

Many commercially made cosmetic products contain *carcinogens*. Even commercially produced natural products can contain harmful chemicals. Some natural ingredients, such as lanolin, a by-product of wool, can accidentally contain chemicals if the sheep were exposed while they were grazing in the pasture. The chemicals can later show up in the lanolin.

BEAUTY BIT

A **carcinogen** is a cancer-causing chemical. A few common carcinogens are diethanolamine (DEA), triethanolamine (TEA), bronopel, dioxane, and colorants Blue 1 and Green 3. Many "natural" products contain ingredients that are known carcinogens or that can combine with other ingredients to form a carcinogen, such as triclosan, benzethonium chloride, formaldehyde, butylated hydroxyanisole, butylated hydroxytoluene, cocamidopropyl betaine, DEA/TEA, PEG, parabens, and dimethicone, just to name a few. Always read labels.

Many common items found in most households can be harmful to humans and pets. Toothpaste, shampoo, antibaterial soap, childen's bubble bath—just to name a few— can, and often do, contain harmful chemicals such as sodium lauryl sulfate (SLS) and preservatives such as formaldehyde (a.k.a. quaternium-15).

Start reading labels. And just because it says "natural" doesn't mean the product is actually natural and safe. Now you see why it's such a good idea to learn to make your own? When you make your own cosmetics, using natural ingredients, you not only help yourself but you also help the environment.

Cleanliness Counts

Now let's discuss where you'll be working and the equipment you'll be using. These are almost as important, healthwise, as the ingredients you'll use.

Sanitize, Sanitize, Sanitize

The surfaces of your kitchen counters and equipment you use when making beauty products may *look* clean, but in truth, they're covered with contaminants. Before you start any project, first thoroughly clean your workspace and all your supplies to ensure everything is free of germs and bacteria that could contaminate your beauty products. Even if you're only making them for yourself, you still need to clean before you start. Sanitize *everything* you'll be using: utensils, mixer beaters, saucepans, containers, counters—*everything*.

> **SAFETY FIRST**
>
> If you don't sanitize your workspace and everything you'll be using, harmful germs, bacteria, mold, and fungus will grow in your products. The bacteria and germs can cause serious infections, and the fungus and mold are just plain nasty and ruin whatever they get into. Never underestimate the importance of cleaning your supplies!

You can still kill the germs and bacteria on your counters and be green while doing it by using white distilled vinegar. Wipe down all the hard surfaces that will come in contact with your project. You can also use regular alcohol. Either one is just fine. You also have a choice of many commercially made antibacterial cleaners, but be aware of what you're actually using. Read the labels before making your choice.

We can't say this enough: it's very important that you sanitize your containers. And sometimes it seems there are as many methods of sterilization as there are home-crafters! Many have tried pouring boiling water into bottles and jars only to stand there and watch them warp from the heat of the water. Some have tried steaming the bottles and jars, and again, watched them warp. Not good.

The simplest and safest way to sanitize your containers is to either use a commercial sanitizer or plain ol' alcohol. Either way will get the job done. No matter which method you choose to use, let the bottles and jars air-dry afterward.

To use alcohol to sanitize your jars and bottles, simply put a small amount of alcohol in the bottle or jar, screw on the lid, and shake. Pour out the alcohol, turn the jar/bottle and lid upside down on a sanitized counter, and let air-dry. You can also use a spray bottle filled with alcohol to spray the lids or small jars. Again, let them air-dry.

Good Sanitizing Products to Use

Let's take a look at some of the many options you have when it comes to sanitizers:

Alcohol You can use regular alcohol and a cloth or gauze to wipe all the counters, equipment, and utensils. Let them air-dry. While you're making beauty products, it's a good idea to keep a spray bottle full of alcohol handy. You may need to spray a spoon or spatula as you work. You can get this alcohol at any drugstore or grocery store.

Hydrogen peroxide   At 3 percent, this peroxide is strong enough to kill most types of bacteria in about 10 minutes. And it's easy to use and readily available at most drugstores. Simply pour a small amount of peroxide onto the counter surface or wipe it on with a cloth or gauze. Hydrogen peroxide is a good option to use as a rinsing substance for sanitized items. Water contains all sorts of contaminants, so it would defeat the sanitizing.

Bleach   You can make the cheapest and most readily available sanitizing solution by adding 1 tablespoon bleach to 1 gallon water. Add your equipment to the mixture, let soak for 20 minutes, and drain. Rinsing supposedly isn't necessary at this concentration, but many home-crafters, myself included, rinse with some boiled water that's been allowed to cool to be sure no off-flavors from the chlorine make it to the final beauty product.

Commercial Sanitizers

Many commercial sanitizers are available online or at specialty stores. Follow the manufacturer's recommendations for using these. Our choice of commercial sanitizers is called One Step. It's easy to work with and requires no rinsing.

Other sanitizers include B-Brite, C-Brite, PBW, Star San, and Iodophor.

> **PRETTY POINTER**
>
> Sanitizing your containers is a boring job, so you could sanitize everything ahead of time, all at once, and store the clean bottles, jars, lids, etc. in zipper-lock bags until you're ready to use them.

Preserving Safety

Washing your hands before and during your projects is also very important. However, no matter how careful you are and how hard you try, sometimes things grow anyway. To avoid this, use an across-the-board preservative or a preservative system.

An across-the-board preservative also kills, mold, fungus, and gram-positive and gram-negative bacteria. You can choose from several on the market, and the type you need depends on the product you're making. (See Appendix E to help you make the correct choice.)

If you decide to start selling your products, you also need to have them tested regularly to ensure they're safe for use.

Caring for Your Skin

Okay. Now that that's all out of the way, let's talk about your skin. After all, that's a big part of how you choose your beauty products, to either make your skin look good or cover what doesn't look good.

In this book, we give you what you need to know to make a full regimen of facial care products, including cleansers, toners, moisturizers, eye gels, night creams, and facial masks. Then we move on to making makeup, with chapters that tell you how to make foundations, concealers, color correctors, blushes, bronzers, eye shadows, eyeliners, and lipsticks.

Even with all those tools at our disposal, and although we all want to look the best we can, we may not know what to do to take care of our skin properly. And even when we do know, we don't always take the time to do what's necessary! It helps to have healthy, youthful genes, but many of us just aren't that lucky.

By following some easy tips, you can have healthier skin that will keep you looking younger and more beautiful for longer. All you have to do is make it a daily habit. Set aside a certain time that's just your time to pamper *you*. Soon you'll look forward to this time!

> **PRETTY POINTER**
>
> When drying your face with a towel, blot, don't rub. And never pull downward on your face. It will fall downward soon enough—don't help speed up the process!

When you get up each morning, wash your face with either a gentle facial wash or a bar of your own homemade facial soap. (Check out our companion book, *The Complete Idiot's Guide to Making Natural Soaps,* for some recipes!) The soap you buy at the store is too harsh for your face, no matter what brand it is.

At night, clean your face with a cleanser so you can remove all your makeup easily.

You can use a toner or astringent to remove any leftover residue from your skin so it's squeaky clean. Be sure to moisturize your skin after you've cleaned it to avoid drying it out. You can make a light moisturizer for summer, and if you need a little more moisturizer in the winter, you can adjust the oils you use to make a heavier version.

You should exfoliate at least two times a week, and three would be better. By doing this, you remove dead skin cells, unclog your pores, and improve the look and feel of your skin. You can create your own facial peels that make your skin feel so good and leave it looking more vibrant and healthy. Facial clay masks also make you feel like you've had a day at the spa. We give you recipes for both in later chapters!

Believe it or not, you can make all these products! The recipes and instructions are in this book, waiting for you to give them a go. With all the recipes we've packed in these pages—over 250 of them!—you could stay busy pampering yourself for at least a year!

And perhaps the best thing about this is that all these recipes use natural ingredients, and therefore won't pollute the air, the earth, or your skin. Now that's living beautiful and beautifully green.

The Least You Need to Know

- Avoiding the potentially dangerous chemicals found in many of today's commercially made beauty products is one very good reason for making your own.
- You have to sanitize everything you plan on using when making beauty products, as well as clean your workspace, but you can do this and still be earth friendly.
- Put your best skin forward by taking good care of it. Make it a routine, and it will soon become one you look forward to every morning and night.

Beautiful Butters and Oils

In This Chapter

- All about butters
- Oils you'll want to get to know
- The best butters and oils for what ails ya

This chapter is filled with butters and oils you can use to make your own natural beauty products. The list might seen long and intimidating, but if you start experimenting with some oils and butters by following the recipes in Part 2, you'll soon become more familiar with what different oils and butters do and can even start creating your own concoctions. And that's where some of the real fun begins!

A Few Notes on Butters and Oils

Before we dive into the list of butters and oils, let's get a few things straight about what you'll see in the following sections. Let's start with the name(s). The first name of a butter or an oil is its common name. Following that is the botanical name. You'll need the botanical name when you start making labels for your beauty products.

You'll see that many of the butters in this list have a hardness value listed. The higher the number, the harder the butter is. You can use the harder butters to thicken lotions and creams.

A shelf life is also listed with each butter and oil. This is the approximate life span of each butter or oil, from the time you open it to when it starts to go rancid. You can lengthen the shelf life of oils. One way is by adding rosemary oleoresin extract (ROE). Simply add 1 tablespoon (14.8 milliliters) per 7 pounds (3.18 kilograms) oil. Be sure to add the extract to the oils as soon as you get them. You can't add the resin to butters, so it might be best to freeze them if you want to keep them longer. Freeze in zipper-lock bags at least 4mm thick, and be sure the butter is double bagged. When ready to use, just set out what you need to thaw.

The properties of the oils and butters are listed when known. This information includes vitamins and minerals that are beneficial to the skin. Some of the uses are listed with each oil and butter so you can get a better idea of what you could use them in.

Butters and Oils for Making Beauty Products

And now, without further ado, here are the butters and oils you can use when making your natural beauty products.

IN THE MIRROR

There are only a few natural butters. The rest are manmade or "designer" butters. The latter are made by hydrogenating the oil. This is a process wherein the oil molecules are forced back into themselves. This creates a very soft butter. Olive butter is an example of one of these designer butters.

Açai oil (*Euterpe Oleracea* pulp oil)   Açai oil contains essential fatty acids; omega-3, -6, and -9; vitamins B_1, B_2, B_3, E, and C; iron; calcium; potassium; amino acids; phytoster; and polyphenols. It helps with anti-aging, dry skin, mature skin, acne, eczema, psoriasis, and muscle aches. Try it in lip products, after-sun products, lotions, facial creams, body butters, and balms. It has a shelf life of 6 months to a year.

Açai oil is pretty new to our market and still very expensive. This oil is being tested for use in fighting cancer and other diseases as well as for weight loss. Many people use the berries to make drinks and shakes.

Almond (sweet) oil (*Prunus Amygdalus*)   Sweet almond oil contains essential fatty acids and vitamins A, B_1, B_2, B_6, and E. It helps with dry and itchy skin, mature skin, eczema, psoriasis, and inflamed skin. Try it in lotions, creams, balms, lip products, bath and body products, and soaps. It has a shelf life of 6 months to a year.

Sweet almond oil isn't very expensive and is used in many of our bath and body products for its properties as well as price. Sweet almond oil is a soft, light-gold-colored oil.

Andiroba oil (*Carapa Guianensis*)   Andiroba oil is antiviral, antifungal, antibacterial, analgesic, anti-inflammatory, antispasmodic, and insecticidal. It contains essential fatty acids oleic, palmitic, linoleic, and stearic. It helps eczema, psoriasis, and skin fungi, and it prevents head lice. It also repels bugs. Try it in massage oil, lotions, facial creams, hair products, balms, and candles. It has a shelf life of 1 year; refrigerate after opening to extend life.

Andiroba oil absorbs easily into the skin and hair.

Apricot kernel oil (*Prunus Armeniaca*)   Apricot kernel oil contains vitamins A, C, E, and potassium. It helps dry and irritated skin and can be used in lotions, creams, body butters, massage oils, lip products, bath oils, and soaps. It has a shelf life of 6 months to a year.

Apricot kernel oil isn't expensive, so it's often used in bath and body products. Apricot kernel oil offers many skin-loving benefits and is a good choice to use in products for mature skin. It's a beautiful golden-yellow oil.

Argan oil (*Argania Spinosa*)   Argan oil is an antioxidant and is antibacterial, antifungal, analgesic, and anti-inflammatory. It contains high amounts of vitamin E and vitamin F (alpha-tocopherol), and it hydrates the skin, helps with anti-aging, reduces swelling, increases skin elasticity, and soothes dry skin. Try it in lotions, creams, body butters, and balms. It has a shelf life of 18 months.

Argan oil won't clog pores, so it's good in any product you want to use it in.

Avocado oil (*Persea Gratissima*)   Avocado oil contains vitamins A, B_1, B_2, D, and E; pantothenic acid; protein; lecithin; and fatty acids. It helps with eczema, psoriasis, scars, and dryness, and it hydrates skin. Try it in lotions, creams, body butters, facial creams, balms, bath products, and soaps. It has a shelf life of 12 months.

Avocado oil is inexpensive and easily absorbed and has emollient properties, making it a great choice for products for mature skin. It's wonderful in shampoo bars and gels.

Babassu oil (*Orbignya Oleifera*)   Some people use this oil for moisturizing in their lotions, but 10 percent oleic acid isn't much. In fact, it's the same as coconut oil. This oil is used more in soap-making than in bath and body products. It is one of the three cleansing oils in soap-making and boosts lather. Babassu oil has a shelf life of 1 or 2 years.

Baobab oil (*Adansonia Digitata*)   Baobab oil contains vitamins A, D, E, and F (alpha-tocopherol). It helps with eczema and psoriasis and moisturizes the skin and hair. Try it in lotions, face creams, body butters, and hair conditioners. It has a shelf life of 2 years.

Baobab oil leaves a silky, smooth feeling and won't clog pores.

Black cumin seed oil (*Nigella Sativa*)   Black cumin seed oil is anti-inflammatory, antibacterial, antiviral, antifungal, and also a parasiticide. It contains protein; carbohydrates; essential fatty acids; vitamins A, B_1, B_2, and C; niacin; and several minerals, including calcium, potassium, iron, magnesium, selenium, and zinc. It also helps relieve muscle pain and earaches. Try it in lotions, skin tonics, balms, and pain creams. It has a shelf life of 6 months. Do refrigerate after opening.

Borage oil (*Borago Officinalis*)   Borage oil is rich in *gamma linolenic acid*, or *GLA*. It helps with eczema, psoriasis, rheumatoid arthritis, sun-damaged skin, dry skin, and repairing damaged hair. Try it in lotions, creams, balms, hair care products, and after-sun products. It has a shelf life of 6 months.

> **BEAUTY BIT**
>
> **Gamma linolenic acid (GLA)** is a polyunsaturated fatty acid, omega-6. It's an antioxidant and helps inflammation.

Buriti oil (*Mauritia Flexuosa*)   Buriti oil contains vitamin E and is a very high source of carotenoids (carrots are, too). It's great for rebuilding, hydrating, and moisturizing the skin, so try it in lotions, creams, and body butters. It has a shelf life of 6 months to 1 year when stored in a cool place.

Buriti oil has a very strong, oily scent and leaves an oily feel to the skin.

Camelina oil (*Camelina Sativa*)   Camelina oil contains essential fatty acids and natural tocopherols. It helps with repairing cells, eczema, psoriasis, improving skin elasticity, and protecting hair. Try it in all types of skin care products, shampoos, and conditioners. It has a shelf life of 2 years.

Camelina oil is good for mature or sensitive skin.

Camellia oil (*Camellia Oleifera*)   Camellia oil is anti-aging. It contains vitamins A, B, and E. It helps moisturize dry skin, fade scars, block UV rays, promote hair growth, and lighten freckles and age spots. It is a carrier oil and can be used for aromatherapy as well. Try it in massage oil, facial creams and lotions, body butters, balms, lip products, and hair and nail care products. It has a shelf life of 2 years.

Canola oil (*Brassica Campestris*)   Canola oil contains oleic and linoleic acid. It's used mainly for moisturizing, so try it in cosmetics, lotions, creams, and soaps. It has a shelf life of up to 1 year.

Cape chestnut oil (*Calodendrum Capense*) Cape chestnut oil, a.k.a. yangu oil, contains essential fatty acids and antioxidants. It helps soften, moisturize, and revitalize skin, and it provides natural UV protection. Try it in facial creams, lotions, hair conditioners, massage oils, balms, and sun care products. It has a shelf life of 1 year. Keep refrigerated after opening for longer shelf life.

Castor oil (*Ricinus Communis*) Castor oil is analgesic, anti-inflammatory, and also a disinfectant. It contains 90 percent ricinoleic acid. It moisturizes skin and promotes healing and pain relief. Try it in cosmetics, lip products, skin and hair care products, sunscreens, perfumes, and both bar and liquid gel soaps. It has a shelf life of 2 years.

IN THE MIRROR

When used in soap-making, castor oil adds conditioning and both creamy and bubbly lather.

Cherry kernel oil (*Prunus Avium*) Cherry kernel oil contains vitamins A and E and is an antioxidant as well as an analgesic. It also contains eleostrearic fatty acid. Cherry kernel oil is great for moisturizing, so try it in lip balms, body butters, moisturizers, creams, and cleansers. It has a shelf life of 1 year.

Cherry kernel oil is similar to sweet almond and peach kernel oil and can be easily substituted for them in formulas. It has a nongreasy feel.

Cocoa butter (*Theobroma Cacao*) Cocoa butter contains natural antioxidants. It helps with dry or itchy skin, stretch marks, skin elasticity, holding moisture in the skin, easing wrinkles, and fading scars and burn marks. Try it in lotions, creams, balms, body butters, bath products, and soaps. It has a shelf life of up to 5 years.

Cocoa butter is solid at room temperature but quickly melts when it comes in contact with the skin. It is sometimes used to thicken products. You can buy cocoa butter in two forms: natural or deodorized.

Coconut oil, fractionated (*Caprylic/Capric Triglyceride*) Fractionated coconut oil offers everything regular coconut oil offers and more. It remains liquid until a very low temperature. Perfumers often use this oil in place of alcohol as a carrier. It also mixes very well with essential oils. It is colorless and has no odor. Its shelf life is indefinite.

Fractionated coconut oil is ideal for massage oils because it won't stain the sheets and it absorbs quickly into the skin, leaving a soft, silky, nongreasy feel.

Coffee oil, green (*Coffea Arabica*)   This oil is abstracted from beans that have not been roasted. It contains fatty acids and sterols. It's also an antioxidant. Coffee oil is good for dry and sensitive skin, mature skin, damaged hair, chapped lips, eczema, and psoriasis. Try it in hair conditioners, lip products, creams, lotions, balms, and hot oil treatments. It has a shelf life of 2 years.

Coffee oil, roasted (*Coffea Arabica*)   Roasted coffee oil is the same as green coffee oil, except the beans have been roasted. It's used the same as green coffee oil and is also often used in aromatherapy and to scent lotions, creams, and other bath and body products. It has a shelf life of 2 years.

Cranberry seed oil (*Vaccinium Macrocarpon*)   Cranberry seed oil is rich in vitamin E; vitamin A; and omega-3, -6, and -9 fatty acids. It helps with dry and itchy skin, eczema, and psoriasis. Try it in lotions, creams, under-eye creams, balms, and lip products. It has a shelf life of 2 years.

Cranberry seed oil is used in many anti-aging facial creams and lotions. It protects the skin cells from damage caused by free radicals and is also useful in hair care products to moisturize the hair and scalp and strengthen the hair.

Cucumber seed oil (*Cucumis Sativus*)   Cucumber seed oil is anti-aging. It contains vitamin E, omega-3, omega-6, and oleic and palmitic acids. It helps with dry hair, brittle nails, acne, eczema, and psoriasis and diminishes wrinkles and stretch marks. Try it in lip products, massage oil, sunscreen products, after-sun products, lotions, creams, facial masks, and balms. It has a shelf life of 1 or 2 years. Refrigeration lengthens its shelf life.

Emu oil   Emu oil is anti-inflammatory, nonirritating, antimicrobial, and hypoallergenic. It's a carrier oil, and its healing properties help with inflamed skin; reducing wrinkles, scars, and stretch marks; moisturizing dry skin; rashes; eczema and psoriasis; painful muscles; and stimulating skin, hair, and nail growth. Try it in lotions, creams, salves, and balms. It has a short shelf life, so be sure to always keep refrigerated.

Emu oil penetrates deep into the skin tissue and is excellent as a carrier oil to bring other ingredients deep into the skin tissue.

IN THE MIRROR

Meadowfoam seed oil is often used in place of emu oil for those who oppose using animal products.

Evening primrose oil (*Oenothera Biennis*)   Evening primrose oil contains omega-6. It helps with dry skin, itchy skin, rosacea, acne, and atopic dermatitis and is good for mature skin. Try it in lotions, facial creams, body butters, and balms. It has a shelf life of 6 to 12 months.

Flaxseed oil (linseed)   Flaxseed oil is anti-aging and contains essential fatty acids palmitic, oleic, and linoleic. It also contains omega-3 and linolenic acid. It's good for mature skin and helps with wrinkles, rosacea, acne, eczema, and psoriasis. Try it in facial scrubs, serums, and soaps. It has a shelf life of up to 1 year. Be sure to refrigerate after opening.

Flaxseed oil is very fragile and must be blended with stable oils or an antioxidant such as rosemary resin extract oil at the rate of .1 percent.

Grapeseed oil (*Vitis Vinifera*)   Grapeseed oil, a by-product of wine-making, contains antioxidants, vitamin E, tocopherols, and essential fatty acid linoleic. It helps with dry and itchy skin, varicose veins, eczema, psoriasis, and acne. Try it in lotions, creams, balms, bath products, and soaps. It has a shelf life of 6 months.

Grapeseed oil is inexpensive, which makes it even more desirable for use in bath and body products!

Hemp seed oil (*Cannabis Sativa*) and hemp seed butter   Hemp seed oil is rich in vitamins A and E, essential fatty acids, and protein. It helps with dry or irritated skin, dry hair, dry scalp, skin lesions, and inflamed skin. Try it in hair care products, lotions, creams, body butters, balms, and soaps. It has a shelf life of 6 months to 1 year. Hydrogenating this oil into a butterlike substance increases the shelf life.

Illipe butter (*Shorea Stenoptera*)   Illipe butter contains essential fatty acids palmitic, oleic, linoleic, and stearic. It helps with moisturizing mature skin, protects skin from losing moisture, and helps heal dry or brittle hair and sunburn. Try it in lotions, creams, body butters, lip products, and balms. It's especially good in foot creams. It has a shelf life of 2 years.

Illipe butter is often substituted for cocoa butter.

Jojoba oil (*Simmondsia Chinensis*)   Jojoba oil contains fatty alcohols; essential fatty acids oleic, eicosenoic, and docosenoic; and omega-9. It stabilizes other oils; binds cosmetic powders; and helps with dry skin, wrinkles, acne, removing eye makeup, and hydrating hair and itchy or dry scalp. Try it in lotions, lipsticks, cosmetics, creams, scrubs, balms, and shower gels. It has an infinite shelf life and can be added to short-life oils to extend their shelf life.

IN THE MIRROR

Jojoba oil is actually a liquid wax and makes a wonderful eye makeup remover. It completely removes mascara and leaves the skin around your eyes well moisturized.

Karanja oil (*Pongamia Glabra*)   Karanja oil is antiseptic and an insecticide. It helps with biliousness, eye ailments, itchiness, leucoderma (vitiligo), rheumatism, skin diseases, wounds, worms, head lice, fleas, and repelling insects. Try it in sprays, lotions, soaps, salves, and balms. It has a shelf life of 2 years.

Use karanja oil full strength or diluted with sesame oil and fragrance on exposed skin for outdoor protection. Bugs do not like the smell!

Kiwi seed oil (*Actinidia Chinensis*)   Kiwi seed oil is anti-aging and contains vitamins C and E, omega-3 fatty acids, potassium, and magnesium. It helps with moisturizing dry skin, eczema, psoriasis, brittle hair, aging skin, and dry lips. Try it in anti-aging creams and lotions, eye creams, lip products, salves, balms, hair conditioners, and makeup removers. It has a shelf life of 1 year, or longer if refrigerated.

Kokum butter (*Garcinia Indica*)   Kokum butter contains vitamin E and essential fatty acids oleic, palmitic, linoleic, and stearic. It helps with dry skin. Try it in balms, body butters, and creams. It has a shelf life of 2 years.

Kokum butter is often used in soap-making to add hardness to the bars.

Kukui oil (*Aleurites Moluccana*)   Kukui oil contains vitamins A, C, and E, and essential fatty acids. It helps with mature skin, acne, scars, wounds, sun- and windburns, eczema, psoriasis, damaged skin, dry or brittle hair, and flaky scalp. Try it in massage oils, lotions, creams, balms, scalp treatment oils, salves, after-sun products, and hair conditioners. It has a shelf life of 1 year if refrigerated.

Kukui oil is nongreasy and easily absorbs into the skin. It's an expensive oil but is worth every penny. I highly recommend this oil for cancer patients to rehydrate their skin.

Lanolin   Lanolin contains cholesterol, esters of fatty acids, and molecular alcohols. It helps with dry, chapped skin, so try it in lipsticks, lotions, and creams. It has a shelf life of 3 years.

Lanolin is a wax, not a fat or oil. It also forms an emulsion with water that's easily absorbed by the skin. In lipstick, lanolin helps the color stick to the lips. Lanolin is very thick and sticky.

Macadamia oil (*Macadamia Integrifolia*)   Macadamia oil contains a high amount of monounsaturated fatty acids. It helps with regeneration of the skin, sunburns, scars, wounds, irritated skin, fine lines, and softening the skin. Try it in lotions, creams, body butters, shaving creams, balms, massage oils, and lip products. It has a shelf life of 1 or 2 years.

Mango butter (*Mangifera Indica*)   Mango butter contains antioxidants, fatty acids, and stearic acid. It helps with dry, chapped skin; eczema; and psoriasis. Try it in body butters, creams, lotions, salves, balms, and soaps. It has a shelf life of 2 or 3 years.

Manketti oil (*Ricinodendron Rautanenii*)   Manketti oil is rich in nutrients and is an antioxidant. It contains vitamin C and eleostrearic acid and is great for sun protection and hair care. Try it in lotions, creams, balms, body butters, shampoos and conditioners, and sun protection products. It has a shelf life of 1 year.

Maracuja oil (*Passiflora Incarnata*)   Maracuja oil is anti-inflammatory, antispasmodic, and antibacterial and contains vitamins A, B, and C. It helps dry and sensitive skin, eczema, psoriasis, dry hair, and dermatitis, and also relieves pain and balances sebum. Try it in lip care products, hair conditioners, lotions, creams, balms, and hot oil treatments. It has a shelf life of 1 year.

PRETTY POINTER

Maracuja oil is good for mature or sensitive skin.

Marula oil (*Sclerocarya Birrea*)   Marula oil contains fatty acids oleic, linoleic, alpha-linolenic, palmitic, and arachidonic. It is an antioxidant and contains tocopherols, sterols, and flavonoids. It helps with conditioning and moisturizing the hair and scalp. Marula oil is often added to cosmetics, such as eye shadows, for its moisturizing properties. Try it in hair treatments, conditioners, lotions, body butters, eye shadows, and lip treatments. It has a shelf life of 1 year. Refrigeration extends its shelf life.

Marula oil is easily absorbed into the skin.

Meadowfoam seed oil (*Limnanthes Alba*)   Meadowfoam seed oil contains fatty acids and is an antioxidant. It is a scent binder and a carrier oil; extends the shelf life of other oils; and helps with moisturizing, UV protection, reducing wrinkles, chapped lips, and damaged hair. Try it in lotions; creams; salves; body butters; shaving creams; hot oil hair conditioners; pain creams; and really any and all bath and body products, hair products, and cosmetics. It has an infinite shelf life.

Meadowfoam seed oil is a nongreasy oil. When blended with shorter shelf life oils, their shelf life is extended. Meadowfoam seed oil penetrates deep into body tissues, so it makes a wonderful carrier oil to deliver other ingredients. You can use meadowfoam in place of emu or ostrich oil in pain creams.

Moringa seed oil (*Moringa Oleifera*)   Also called ben oil, moringa seed oil is said to be antiseptic and anti-inflammatory. It contains vitamins A and C and fatty acids oleic, palmitic, stearic, and behenic. It helps with moisturizing and conditioning. Try it in lotions, creams, balms, body butters, and hair care products. It has a shelf life of up to 5 years.

Mowrah butter (*Madhuca Latifolia*)   Mowrah butter contains essential fatty acids oleic, palmitic, linoleic, and stearic. It helps heal and moisturize burns and dry, chapped skin. Try it in lotions, creams, body butters, balms, salves, and lip products. It has a shelf life of 1 year.

Mowrah butter has wonderful healing properties. It gives your lotions, creams, lip balms, and lipsticks a lovely creamy feeling.

IN THE MIRROR

Recently mowrah butter has become very difficult to buy due to bad crop output. I have found the "gently" refined version but not the ultra refined, which I prefer to use.

Neem seed oil (*Azadirachta Indica*)   Neem seed oil is antiseptic, antifungal, antibacterial, antiviral, and dermatological, and an analgesic and insecticide. It helps with fleas, lice, wounds, and insect stings. Try it in shampoos, salves, and sprays. It has a shelf life of 2 years.

Neem seed oil kills fleas and head lice but is nontoxic to humans and animals, and therefore very safe to use on children and pets. You can also use neem cakes in your garden to keep out ground bugs. Mix neem seed oil with water to spray your plants.

PRETTY POINTER

By adding neem seed oil to shampoo, you have a kid-friendly, lice-killing shampoo that's a safer way to kill the lice without using a commercially prepared insecticide product. Add 15 to 20 drops of neem seed oil to 2 ounces of your regular shampoo.

Olive oil (*Olea Europaea*)   Olive oil contains monounsaturated fat, vitamin E, phenols, and omega-3 and -6 fatty acids. It helps with wrinkles; dry, brittle hair and nails; and mature or sensitive skin. Try it in lotions, creams, and balms. It has a shelf life of 1 year.

This oil is one of the base oils soap-makers use.

Olive oil pomace   Olive oil pomace works a lot like jojoba, shea, or kukui nut oil and can retain moisture in the skin without blocking the skin's ability to breathe. Products in the olive oil family are great to use in many bath and body products, not just for soap! Olive oil pomace is very good for mature, sensitive skin. It's even reported to be a disinfectant and to have wound-healing properties. It has a shelf life of 1 year.

Ostrich oil   Ostrich oil contains omega-3, -6, and -9 fatty acids; vitamin E; and amino acids. It helps heal dry skin, rheumatoid pain, dermatitis, eczema, psoriasis, burns, and bed sores. Try it in salves, lotions, creams, and balms. Be sure to keep this one refrigerated; it has a shelf life of 12 to 18 months, longer if frozen.

There isn't a lot of difference between emu and ostrich oil.

IN THE MIRROR

The Romans and Egyptians regularly used ostrich oil to moisturize their skin. Cleopatra is said to have used ostrich oil.

Palm oil (*Elaeis Guineensis*)   Palm oil comes from the meat of the fruit and contains saturated and unsaturated fats. It's mainly used for moisturizing. Palm oil separates like milk and has to be completely melted and then stirred before each use. Try it in lotions, creams, and balms. It has a shelf life of 2 years.

Bleached and deodorized palm oil is widely used for soap-making as the base oil because of its stability. It is solid in cool or cold temperatures.

Palm oil, red unrefined   Red palm oil contains two of the most important types of vitamin E and a high amount of carotene. It helps with dry skin, wrinkles, and general moisturizing. Try it in lotions, creams, scrubs, balms, lip products, and soaps. It has a shelf life of 2 years.

In Africa, red palm oil is the main cooking oil. Red palm oil separates, but because it's a hard oil, you can't just stir it to mix. You'll have to first melt the entire container and then stir it well before use. Sometimes you can find red palm *butter*, which is actually homogenized red palm oil. This is much easier to work with because it won't separate. When you use red palm oil, all your products will have a soft apricot/yellow color. Some people like the color and some don't.

Papaya seed oil (*Carica Papaya*)   Papaya seed oil contains omega-3 and -6 essential fatty acids. It helps with dry skin, dry or brittle hair, wrinkles, acne, eczema, and psoriasis. Try it in lotions, creams, hair conditioners, and hot oil treatments. It has a shelf life of 2 years.

Passion fruit oil (*Passiflora Incarnate*)   Passion fruit oil contains vitamins A, B, and C. It helps with acne and strengthening skin tissue. Try it in facial washes, lotions, creams, balms, salves, and cosmetics. It has a shelf life of 1 or 2 years.

Peach kernel oil (*Prunus Persica*)   Peach kernel oil contains vitamins A, B, and E. It is a carrier oil and helps with dry or mature skin. It soaks quickly into the skin, leaving the skin feeling soft and moisturized. Try it in lotions, creams, balms, and cosmetics. It's also great for massage oils and aromatherapy use. It has a shelf life of 2 years.

Peach kernel oil is nongreasy.

Peanut oil (*Arachis Hypogaea*)   Peanut oil contains vitamin E. It helps with dry and mature skin, eczema, and psoriasis. Try it in lotions, creams, and soaps. It has a shelf life of 6 months to 1 year.

> **SAFETY FIRST**
>
> If you use peanut oil in any of your products, be sure to label it clearly so anyone with a peanut allergy will know not to use it.

Pequi oil (*Caryocar Braziliensis*)   Pequi oil is anti-aging and contains vitamin A. It helps with dry skin, eczema, psoriasis, frizzy and brittle hair, and general moisturizing. Try it in lotions, creams, balms, salves, hair conditioners, and hot oil treatments. It has a shelf life of 2 years.

Perilla seed oil (*Perilla Ocymoides*)   Perilla seed oil contains omega-3 fatty acids and is an antiseptic. It helps with acne, so try it in facial creams, lotions, scrubs, and balms. It has a shelf life of 1 or 2 years.

Pomegranate seed oil (*Punica Granatum*)   Pomegranate seed oil is anti-inflammatory and is an antioxidant. It contains fatty acids oleic, palmitic, linolenic, punicic, and stearic. It's good for moisturizing dry skin, helps with skin elasticity, and balances skin pH. Try it in facial lotions and creams, body lotions, body butters, and balms. It has a shelf life of 6 months to 1 year, and longer if kept refrigerated.

Poppy seed oil (*Papaver Somniferum*)   Poppy seed oil contains essential fatty acids linoleic, oleic, and palmitic. Use in hair care products, creams, and balms. It has a shelf life of 5 months to 1 year, or longer if kept refrigerated.

Poppy seed oil contains similar properties to hemp seed oil and can be used as a substitute.

Pumpkin seed oil (*Cucurbita Pepo*)   Pumpkin seed oil contains omega-3 and -6 fatty acids; vitamins A, C, and E; and zinc. It helps with rosacea, eczema, psoriasis, burns, wounds, and scars. Try it in lotions, creams, salves, and balms. It has a shelf life of 1 year.

Unrefined pumpkin seed oil is a very dark color, while the refined oil is almost clear. This oil is very rich, so a little goes a long way in your products.

Red raspberry seed oil (*Rubus Idaeus*)   Red raspberry seed oil contains vitamins A and E and omega-3 and -6 fatty acids. It is anti-inflammatory and helps with dry skin, eczema, psoriasis, and sun protection. Try it in lotions, creams, lip products, and balms. It has a shelf life of 2 years.

Red raspberry seed oil can also be used to extend the shelf life of other oils when mixed in.

Rice bran oil (*Oryza Sativa*)   Rice bran oil contains gamma oryzanol. It's good for moisturizing and for use in infusing herbs. Try it in lotions, under-eye creams, cleansing creams, and baby products. It has a shelf life of 1 year.

Rice bran oil feels nice on the skin and is very mild. It's an excellent moisturizer and gives soothing protection to skin.

Rosehip seed oil (*Rosa Rubiginosa*)   Rosehip seed oil contains fatty acids and has anti-aging properties. It renews skin cells, repairs damaged tissue, fades age spots, and helps with eczema and general moisturizing. Try it in facial lotions, creams, and soaps. It has a shelf life of 12 to 18 months if refrigerated.

IN THE MIRROR

Rosehip seed oil is pressed from wild roses. It is an excellent choice to use in your eczema and anti-aging products.

Safflower oil, high oleic (*Carthamus Tinctorius*)   High oleic safflower oil contains vitamin E (tocopherols, essential fatty acids oleic, palmitic, and linoleic). It also contains lecithin and carotenoids. It helps moisturize dry skin and hair, so try it in creams, lotions, hair conditioners, and balms. It has a shelf life of 2 years.

This would be a great addition to all your body products. If you don't have the high oleic type of safflower oil, be sure to add rosemary oleo resin to extend its shelf life. It is also said that this oil used in your diet will help get rid of belly fat.

Sal butter (*Shorea Robusta*)   Sal butter contains fatty acids oleic, palmitic, linoleic, and stearic. It softens and moisturizes skin and promotes healing from sun and wind damage. Try it in stick balms, lotions, body butters, and soaps. It has a shelf life of 1 year.

Sal butter is very stable and won't go rancid quickly.

Sesame seed oil (*Sesamum Indicum*)   Sesame seed oil contains vitamins A and E, plus several essential proteins. It is antibacterial, antioxidant, and antifungal. It helps heal dry skin, psoriasis, dry scalp, dandruff, skin fungi, athlete's foot, acne, mild scrapes and cuts, and diaper irritation. Try it in facial washes, shower gels, lotions, creams, salves, balms, conditioners, and massage oils. It has a shelf life of 1 year.

Sesame seed oil is resistant to clouding at low temperatures.

Shea butter (*Butyrospermum Parkii*)   Shea butter contains vitamins A, E, and F and is anti-inflammatory and antimicrobial. It helps with dry skin, burns, sores, scars, dermatitis, psoriasis, eczema, dandruff, and stretch marks. Try it in lotions, creams, body butters, shaving creams, lip products, and soaps. It has a shelf life of 1 or 2 years but will last longer if refrigerated. It can also be frozen.

Shea butter is easily absorbed into the skin and does not clog pores. It can help protect against the sun's UV rays. Shea butter can be used in just about all bath and body products.

IN THE MIRROR

The extraction process for shea butter can be quite time-consuming. It can take 20 to 30 hours to extract just 2 pounds of shea butter!

Strawberry oil (*Fragaria Anassa*)   Strawberry oil contains vitamins A, E, and F, and omega-3 and -4 fatty acids. It has anti-aging properties and helps with fine lines and dry skin. Try it in creams, lotions, salves, balms, and body butters. It has a shelf life of 2 years.

Strawberry oil is easily absorbed into the skin and has a light, pleasant fragrance.

Sunflower oil, high oleic (*Helianthus Annuus*)   High oleic sunflower oil contains vitamins A, D, and E as well as essential fatty acids. It soothes and moisturizes skin and won't clog pores. Try it in creams, lotions, baby products, balms, and soaps. It has a shelf life of 2 years.

This is our favorite oil for infusing herbs.

Tamanu oil (*Calophyllum Inophyllum*)   Tamanu oil is antibacterial, antifungal, and anti-inflammatory and an antioxidant. It contains essential fatty acids oleic, palmitic, linoleic, and stearic. Its healing properties help with skin ulcers, rashes, boils, cuts, sores, acne, scars, ringworm, athlete's foot, diabetic sores, diaper rash, insect bites, and psoriasis. Try in salves and balms, and even by itself. It has a shelf life of 6 months to 1 year.

Tucuma butter (*Astrocaryum Tucuma*)   Tucuma butter is an antioxidant. It contains vitamin A and essential fatty acids omega-3, -6, and -9. Try it in creams, lotions, body butters, conditioners, masks, hair care products, and lip products. It has a shelf life of 2 years from its production date.

Turkey red oil (*Sulfated Ricinus Communis*)   Turkey red oil, which gets its name from its red color, contains triglycerides and fatty acids. It's the same as castor oil except it hasn't been refined. Add this oil to your bath oils and bath bombs. It has a shelf life of 2 years.

This is the only oil that will completely disperse in water. That means that when used in bath products, the oil will combine with the water in the tub and won't leave an oily residue or ring in the bathtub.

Ucuuba butter (*Virola Sebifera L.*)   Ucuuba butter, which is so dark it looks black, contains essential fatty acids. It repels insects and helps with dry skin. Try it in black soap, balms, and lotions. It has a shelf life of 2 years from its production date.

Walnut oil (*Juglans Regia*)   Walnut oil has great anti-aging properties. It helps soothe and moisturize skin, is good for mature skin, and smoothes wrinkles and fine lines. Try it in anti-aging products, those for mature skin, lip balms, eye creams, and lotions. It has a shelf life of 1 year.

PRETTY POINTER

Use walnut oil at 10 to 15 percent of total product weight in anti-aging and skin-toning products.

Watermelon oil (*Citrullus Vulgaris*)   Watermelon oil, also called kalahari oil, is a stable oil that's very light in texture. It contains essential fatty acids oleic and linoleic plus zinc and iron. It is also a carrier oil. Watermelon oil helps balance the oil the skin produces, making it a good ingredient to use in formulations for those with oily skin. It does not clog pores. Try it in hair care products, facial creams, lotions, baby products, and body butters. Its shelf life is indefinite.

Watermelon oil can restore elasticity to the skin. All skin types can use it. It is not greasy at all, yet it is very moisturizing.

Wheat germ oil (*Triticum Vulgare*)   Wheat germ oil contains vitamins A, D, and E. It helps with dry skin, eczema, dermatitis, wrinkles, and fine lines. Try it in facial creams and lotions, lip products, body creams and lotions, balms, and body butters. It has a shelf life of 1 year.

The Least You Need to Know

- Learning about different oils helps you formulate your own products. Before you know it, you will be formulating like a pro!
- Choosing which butters or oils you want to use can be a challenge, but with a little knowledge of what each butter or oil does, your decision-making is easier.
- Have certain needs? You can find an oil or butter that is best for them.

All About Essential Oils

In This Chapter

- Skin-soothing essential oils
- Scenting your home and your favorite lotions, creams, and soaps
- Going green with cleansing essential oils

Essential oils have many uses. You can use them in air fresheners, bath products, candles, creams and lotions, foot baths, hair care products, massage oil, room air disinfectants and vaporizers, and more. They're even used in many beauty products!

When MRSA and other super bugs came on the health scene recently, many people became very worried. But after much research, there seems to be information on essential oils being used to stop dangerous germs some 65 years ago. It seems that different bacteria and viruses can become resistant to medicine, but essential oils have so many different properties, bacteria cannot become resistant to them.

Not only can you use an essential oil spray to rid a room of illness-causing germs, you can also use a diffuser fitted over a lightbulb to infuse the room with the essential oil. Simply put a few drops of the pure essential oil on a diffuser, fit it on the bulb, and the heat of the bulb will evaporate the oil into the room.

Note: The information in this chapter isn't meant to take the place of professional medical help. It's only a guideline of known uses for essential oils.

How Much Essential Oil to Use?

When including essential oils in your beauty products, do not use them as if they were fragrance oils. Because essential oils are distilled from the roots, bark, flower, stems, and leaves of plants, they contain the true essence of the plant they're derived from.

That makes them very potent, and they can be irritating if used in a strong amount. We recommend you don't use more than 2.5 percent of the total finished weight of your recipe.

For example: if the total weight of a batch of cream is 32 ounces (907.2 grams), the most essential oil or blend of essential oils you'd want to use is .8 ounce (22.7 grams).

If you're using essential oils in candles, you can use the recommended amount for the type of candle you're making.

It's also recommended that you don't use essential oils on babies under the age of 3 months, and many of these oils cannot be used on children or pregnant and nursing women at all. Throughout the chapter, we indicate which oils can or cannot be used in these situations.

Essential Oils for Making Beauty Products

Let's take a look at the essential oils you can use when making your natural beauty products.

Anise (*Pimpinella Anisum*)   This brown but sometimes clear essential oil is anti-spasmodic and is commonly used for muscle aches, arthritis, cramps, nervous tension, depression, rheumatism, colds, and flu. It has a clove or licorice scent.

Balsam of Peru (*Myroxylon Pereirae*)   This dark brown essential oil is commonly used in men's colognes and for chapped hands and feet. It relieves the itch of eczema and dermatitis, helps coughing and rashes, and soothes stress. It smells very sweet and earthy.

Basil, sweet (*Ocimum Basilicum*)   This clear essential oil is antispasmodic, anti-inflammatory, *analgesic*, and antibacterial. It's commonly used for sinusitis, colds, flu, coughs, insect bites, and insect repellent. Basil has an herbal scent.

BEAUTY BIT

An **analgesic** reduces or eliminates pain.

Bay laurel (*Laurus Nobilis*)   This clear essential oil is commonly used for aches and pains, sprains, bruises, hair loss, oily hair, dandruff, colds, and flu. Bay laurel has an earthy scent. *Do not use if you are pregnant or nursing.*

Bay rum (*Pimenta Racemosa*)   This dark yellow essential oil is used for aches and pains, sprains, general hair care, dandruff, oily hair, and men's cologne. It has a spicy scent.

Benzoin (*Styrax Benzoin*)   Brown in color, this essential oil is commonly used to help acne, eczema and psoriasis, arthritis, bronchitis, coughing, and dry skin. It has a creamy vanilla scent.

Bergamot (*Citrus Bergamia*)   This essential oil is a yellow-green color. It's antiseptic and antifungal and is commonly used for acne, oily skin conditions, abscesses, boils, cold sores, itching, depression, psoriasis, and stress. Bergamot is a *photo-sensitizer*, which means it reacts with sunlight. Be sure to use the bergaptene-free version. Bergamot has a citrus with a touch of floral scent.

> **BEAUTY BIT**
>
> If an essential oil is a **photo-sensitizer,** it decreases the skin's ability to tolerate ultraviolet light. This can cause itching, inflammation, and burning.

Cajeput (*Melaleuca Leucadendron*)   This light yellow essential oil is antiseptic, antifungal, antiviral, and antibacterial. It's commonly used for acne, coughing, asthma, bronchitis, sinusitis, and aches. This is another melaleuca like tea tree, niaouli, and rosalina. It has a fruity scent.

Camphor (*Cinnamomum Camphora*)   This deep yellow essential oil is analgesic, antiseptic, and antispasmodic. Commonly used for stiff muscles and inflammation, it has a pungent, camphorous scent. *Always use very sparingly. Do not use if you are pregnant, suffer from epilepsy, and/or have asthma. Do not use it on babies.*

Carrot seed (*Daucus Carota*)   This golden yellow essential oil is commonly used to help mature skin and wrinkles, thicken hair, soothe eczema and psoriasis, and help scars. It doesn't smell like carrots! It's earthy and a little harsh.

Cassia (*Cinnamonum Cassia*)   Cassia is a yellow-brown oil most often used for indigestion, colds, flu, and fragrance. It has the sweet woodsy smell of cinnamon. *Do not use on the skin or products for the skin.*

> **SAFETY FIRST**
>
> Do not use cassia (*Cinnamomum Cassia*) in topical blends because it's an irritant and sensitizer. This is one that would be good to use in the diffuser instead. And don't confuse it with cinnamon bark. Cassia, also known as Chinese cinnamon, is a very strong antimicrobial.

Cedarwood, Atlas (*Cedrus Atlantica*)   This light yellow essential oil is commonly used for acne, dandruff, eczema, psoriasis, alopecia, oily skin, oily scalp, oily hair, men's cologne, arthritis, bronchitis, and stress. It has the scent of fresh cedar trees. *Do not use if you are pregnant. Do not use on children.*

Chamomile, German (*Matricaria Recutita*)   A dark blue color, this essential oil is anti-inflammatory and antispasmodic. It's commonly used for eczema; psoriasis; itchy, dry, and flaky skin; boils; wounds; sores; insect bites; dermatitis; arthritis; sprains; and headaches. It has an herbal scent.

Chamomile, Roman (*Anthemis Nobilis*)   This light blue essential oil is anti-inflammatory and antispasmodic. It's commonly used for eczema, psoriasis, dry skin, wounds, sores, boils, insect bites, dermatitis, arthritis, and headaches. It has an herbal scent. *Use this type of chamomile for children and the elderly.*

Cinnamon bark (*Cinnamomum Zeylanicum*)   This yellow-brown essential oil is antibacterial and antifungal. It's commonly used for fragrancing and in room sprays to kill airborne germs, as well as for lice, scabies, and stress. It has a strong, spicy cinnamon scent. *Do not use in topical products.*

Cinnamon bark is much stronger than cinnamon leaf.

Cinnamon leaf (*Cinnamomum Zeylanicum*)   Yellow-brown cinnamon leaf essential oil is a milder version of cinnamon bark essential oil. It's antibacterial and antifungal. Use it in room sprays to kill airborne germs, lice, and scabies, and to ease stress. It smells spicy, just like cinnamon. *Do not use if you are pregnant or nursing.*

Clary sage (*Salvia Sclaria*)   This light yellow essential oil is analgesic and antispasmodic and is commonly used for asthma, coughing, and stress. Clary sage has an earthy herbal scent. *Do not use if you are pregnant or nursing.*

Clove bud (*Eugenia Caryophyllus*)   This yellow-brown essential oil is used for room sprays, men's colognes, sprains, toothaches, asthma, and bronchitis. It has a warm, spicy scent. *Use with caution; it can be irritating to the skin.*

Combava petitgrain (*Citrus Hystrix*)   This very pale yellow essential oil is anti-infectious and antiseptic. It's commonly used for acne and oily skin. It has a woodsy and slightly floral scent. *Do not use on sensitive skin.*

IN THE MIRROR

Twelve essential oils are mentioned in the Bible: cassia, cedarwood, cistus, cypress, frankincense, myrrh, galbanum, hyssop, myrtle, onycha, sandalwood, and spikenard.

Coriander (*Coriandrum Sativum*)   This light yellow essential oil is anti-inflammatory and is commonly used for arthritis, blackheads, oily skin, aches, and fatigue. It has a spicy and woodsy scent.

Cypress (*Cupressus Sempervirens*)   This light yellow essential oil is antiseptic, antispasmodic, and a deodorant. It's commonly used for eczema, varicose veins, and oily skin. Cypress has a woodsy scent.

Elemi (*Canarium Luzonicum*)   This very pale yellow essential oil is antifungal, antiseptic, and analgesic. It's commonly used for warts, dry or mature skin, dermatitis, scars, coughing, wounds, acne, and eczema. Because of its mildness, it would be good to use in deodorants. It has a spicy and citrus scent.

Eucalyptus (*Eucalyptus Globulus*)   This essential oil is clear and has analgesic, antifungal, antiviral, and antibacterial properties. It's commonly used for blackheads, acne, blemishes, cold sores, flu, bronchitis, and sinusitis. It has a camphorous scent. *Never take eucalyptus internally.*

> **PRETTY POINTER**
>
> You can make a candle using eucalyptus essential oil and burn it for 10 minutes to kill all the germs, bacteria, and mold in the air.

Eucalyptus (*Eucalyptus Radiata*)   This almost-clear essential oil is analgesic, antifungal, antiviral, and antibacterial. It's commonly used for room sprays, blackheads, acne, blemishes, cold sores, flu, fever, sinusitis, and bronchitis. This oil has all the therapeutic benefits of *Eucalyptus Globulus* but is a more gentle and pleasant oil to use. Eucalyptus has a strong camphorous scent. *Never take eucalyptus internally.*

Eucalyptus (*Eucalyptus Smithii*)   This very pale yellow essential oil is analgesic, antifungal, antiviral, and antibacterial. It's commonly used for room sprays, blackheads, acne, blemishes, cold sores, flu, bronchitis, and sinusitis. This one is the mildest of all the eucalyptus types and is suggested for use in children. It has a camphorous scent. *Never take eucalyptus internally.*

Eucalyptus, lemon (*Eucalyptus Citriodora*)   This very pale yellow essential oil is analgesic, antifungal, antiviral, and antibacterial. It's commonly used for room sprays, blackheads, acne, blemishes, cold sores, flu, bronchitis, and sinusitis. It's very similar to *Eucalyptus Globulus* and has a camphorous and lemon scent. *Never take eucalyptus internally.*

Fir needle (*Abies Alba*)   This very pale yellow essential oil is analgesic, antiseptic, and a deodorant. It's commonly used for arthritis, bronchitis, flu, colds, and aches. It has a woodsy scent.

Fir needle, Canada (*Abies Canadensis*)   This light yellow essential oil is analgesic, antiseptic, and a deodorant. It's commonly used for arthritis, bronchitis, flu, colds, aches, deodorants, and room sprays. It has a woodsy scent.

Frankincense (*Boswellia Carteri*)   This light yellow essential oil is commonly used for dry and mature skin, wrinkles, blemishes, anxiety, scars, stretch marks, bronchitis, asthma, coughing, and wounds. It has a spicy, balsamic scent.

Galbanum (*Ferula Galbaniflua*)   This clear essential oil is commonly used for inflammation, wounds, dry or mature skin, wrinkles, scars, abscesses, bronchitis, acne, cuts, lice, stretch marks, and muscle aches. It smells very earthy, balsamic, and spicy.

Geranium (*Pelargonium Graveolens*)   This light yellow essential oil, also known as rose geranium, is commonly used for pain relief, wounds, acne, dull skin, lice, menopause, cellulite, and oily skin. It has a floral scent.

Ginger (*Zingiber Officinale*)   This light yellow essential oil is antibacterial and analgesic. It's commonly used for a warming oil, pain relief, muscle aches, and arthritis. It has a very warm earthy and spicy scent.

Grapefruit (*Citrus Paradisi*)   This light yellow essential oil is used for dull skin and to eliminate water weight and cellulite. It has a citrus fragrance.

Helichrysum (*Helichrysum Italicum*)   This light yellow essential oil is antifungal, antiviral, and antibacterial. It's commonly used for scars, acne, dermatitis, abscesses, boils, burns, cuts, wounds, eczema, and irritated skin. It also promotes cell growth. It has an herbal fragrance.

> **PRETTY POINTER**
>
> *Helichrysum Italicum* has become very expensive. A cheaper version, which works just as well, is *Helichrysum Gymnocephalum*.

Jasmine (*Jasminum Grandiflorum*)   This dark brown essential oil is antiseptic and relieves muscle cramps. It's commonly used for dry skin and dermatitis, depression, and sensitive skin, as well as pain and cramping. Jasmine essential oil is very expensive, so use it sparingly. The essential oil smells like the flower.

Juniper berry (*Juniperus Communis*)   This clear essential oil is antiseptic, antispasmodic, and an astringent. It's commonly used for acne, blocked pores, eczema, psoriasis, inflammations, colds, and flu. It has a woodsy scent.

Labdanum (*Cistus Ladaniferus*)   This clear essential oil, also known as rose of Sharon and citrus oil, is antibacterial, antifungal, and antiviral. It's commonly used for wrinkles, mature skin, and room sprays. It has a citrus scent.

Lavender (*Lavandula Officinalis*)   This very light yellow essential oil has all the goodies of the other lavenders. It's analgesic, antispasmodic, antiviral, antibacterial, and antifungal. It's mainly used for inflammations, acne, abscesses, blisters, boils, asthma, muscle aches, lice, strains, sprains, vertigo, dry skin, and eczema and other skin problems. It has an herbal floral scent. *Do not use on children or the elderly.*

Lavender, Bulgarian (*Lavender Angustifolia*)   This very pale yellow essential oil is analgesic, antispasmodic, antiviral, antibacterial, and antifungal. It's commonly used for inflammations, acne, abscesses, blisters, boils, asthma, muscle aches, lice, strains, sprains, vertigo, dry skin, and eczema and other skin problems. This is the lavender I use to make bath oil for my ADHD grandson; it soothes him and helps him sleep. *It is safe enough to use on children and the elderly. Do not use on babies younger than 3 months.*

Lavender, super (*Lavandula Hybrid var. Super French*)   This very light yellow essential oil is antispasmodic and is commonly used for wounds, cuts, bruises, dermatitis, scars, scabies, insect repellent, insect bites, hypertension, depression, headaches, asthma, stretch marks, cramps, allergies, coughing, and sores. It has a floral scent.

Lavendin, grosso (*Lavandula Hybrid var. Grosso French*)   This very light yellow essential oil is antiseptic as well as being a stimulant. It's commonly used for inflammations, acne, abscesses, blisters, boils, asthma, muscle aches, lice, strains, sprains, vertigo, dry skin, and eczema and other skin problems. It has a sweet herbal and floral scent.

Lemon (*Citrus Limonum*)   This dark yellow essential oil is antineuralgic, antirheumatic, antiseptic, antibacterial, insecticidal, and an astringent. It's commonly used for warts, flu, colds, corns, pimples, oily skin, athlete's foot, and varicose veins. It has a lemon fragrance. *Lemon can be a sensitizer.*

Lemongrass (*Cymbopogon Citratus*)   This yellow essential oil is anti-inflammatory. It's commonly used for muscle aches, enlarged pores, oily skin, athlete's foot, insect repellent, stress, and scabies. It has an earthy lemon scent.

Lemongrass, East Indian (*Cymbopogon Flexuosus*)   This yellow essential oil is commonly used for muscle aches, enlarged pores, oily skin, athlete's foot, insect repellent, stress, and scabies. It has an earthy lemon scent.

Lime (*Citrus Aurantifolia*)   This light green essential oil is typically used for men's cologne, colds, flu, asthma, and acne and pimples. It has a fruity lime scent. *Lime can be a sensitizer.*

> **PRETTY POINTER**
>
> Blending lemon and lime essential oils makes a delightful fragrance blend.

Litsea cubeba (*Litsea Cubeba*)   This light yellow essential oil is commonly used for acne, oily skin, and excess sweat. *Do not use straight on the skin; add to a carrier oil.*

Mandarin, red (*Citrus Reticulate*) This green essential oil is antiseptic. It's commonly used for muscle cramps, acne, pimples, wrinkles, scars, and stress. It has a sweet citrus scent.

Manuka (*Leptospermum Scoparium*) This clear essential oil is antibacterial, antifungal, and antiviral. It's typically used for oily skin, insect bites, cuts, sores, athlete's foot, ringworm, colds, flu, sinusitis, itching, cold sores, and pimples. It's similar in properties to tea tree oil and can be substituted for it in formulations. It has been proven effective against both strep and staph infections. Manuka has an earthy, balsamic scent.

Marjoram, Spanish (*Thymus Mastichina*) This light yellow essential oil is analgesic and antiseptic. It's commonly used for muscle cramps, swollen joints, bronchitis, coughing, sprains, and stress. It has an herbal scent.

Marjoram, sweet (*Origanum Majorana*) This pale yellow essential oil is an antiseptic. It's commonly used for muscle cramps, swollen joints, bronchitis, coughing, rheumatism, sprains, and stress. It has an herbal scent. *Do not use if you are pregnant.*

Melissa (*Melissa Officinalis*) This yellow essential oil is useful against various strains of flu virus. It's also used for dermatitis, pimples, infected teeth, room sprays, colognes, insect bites, bronchitis, coughing, depression, insomnia, menstrual cramps, asthma, anxiety, and eczema. It has an herbal scent.

Myrrh (*Commiphora Myrrha*) This brown essential oil is an antiseptic, astringent, disinfectant, and deodorant. It's commonly used for infected teeth, infected gums, eczema, sore throat, athlete's foot, jock itch, ringworm, bronchitis, dry skin, itching, and hemorrhoids. This is the most amazing oil or powder to have around the house. It has an earthy and balsamic fragrance.

IN THE MIRROR

Evidence of herbal perfumes was found in King Tutankhamen's tomb.

Myrtle (*Myrtus Communis*) This light yellow essential oil very similar to eucalyptus is antibacterial, antiseptic, and an astringent. It's commonly used for room sprays, cough, sore throat, and asthma. This is a very mild essential oil that can be used to treat children and the elderly. It has a sweet but camphorous scent.

Neroli (*Citrus Aurantium*) This dark brown essential oil is a deodorant and an antiseptic. It's commonly used for acne, depression, mature skin, scars, stretch marks, stress, and as a muscle relaxant. Because it's so gentle, it's good to use for all skin types. It has a sweet citrus scent.

Niaouli (*Melaleuca Quinquenervia*)   This clear essential oil is commonly used to help oily skin, aches, sore throats, colds, coughing, cuts, stretch marks, scars, bronchitis, and acne. Niaouli is a melaleuca and can be substituted for tea tree oil. It has a harsh earthy and musty scent.

Orange, bitter (*Citrus Sinensis*)   This yellow-orange essential oil is an antiseptic and is commonly used for room sprays, flu, colds, infected gums, stress, and as a local disinfectant. This oil smells like oranges. *Bitter orange is a citrus and can be a sensitizer when used on the skin.*

Oregano (*Origanum Vulgare*)   This light yellow essential oil is an antiseptic. Use it for room sprays and disinfecting surfaces. Oregano has a strong, harsh, herbal scent.

Palmarosa (*Cymbopogon Martini*)   This light yellow essential oil is antifungal and antiviral. It stimulates cellular growth, helps dry skin, and regulates sebum. It has a floral scent. *Do not use if you are pregnant or nursing. Do not use on children or anyone who has medical conditions.*

Patchouli (*Pogostemon Patchouli*)   This dark brown essential oil is an antiseptic, astringent, and deodorant, and is antifungal. It's commonly used for scars, dry skin, acne, eczema, scalp disorders, athlete's foot, dermatitis, oily skin, mature skin, insect repellent, and hair care. Patchouli oil has a sweet earthy and woodsy scent.

Pepper, black (*Piper Nigrum*)   This clear essential oil is analgesic and antiseptic. It's commonly used for muscle aches, arthritis, and muscle cramps. It's also great to use in a massage oil. Black pepper has a spicy peppercorn scent.

Peppermint (*Mentha Piperita*)   This light yellow essential oil has great pain-relieving properties. It can be used for muscle aches, cramps, bruises, joint pain, colic, nausea, asthma, fever, headaches, vertigo, sinusitis, and scabies. Use it in pain cream, room spray, and massage oil. It smells like very strong peppermint. *Do not use if you are pregnant.*

Petitgrain, bigarade (*Citrus Aurantium*)   This light yellow essential oil is an antiseptic and deodorant. Use it as a room spray and to help acne and oily skin. It's made from the leaves of the bitter orange and can be used in place of neroli. It smells earthy and floral.

Petitgrain, clementine (*Citrus Clementine*)   This light yellow essential oil is commonly used for oily skin, acne, and stress. Clementine petitgrain has the same uses and properties of bigarade petitgrain, but has a much softer and sweeter woodsy and citrus scent.

Pine (*Pinus Sylvestris*)   This clear essential oil is antiseptic, antibacterial, and a deodorant. It's commonly used for disinfecting surfaces, cough relief, colds, and flu. It has the woodsy scent of pine trees. *Pine oil can be irritating to the skin.*

Ravensara (*Agathophyllum Aromatica*)   This light yellow essential oil is commonly used along with tamanu (*Calophyllum Inophyllum*) oil for shingles. It smells earthy and woodsy. *Do not use if you are pregnant. Do not use on children.*

Rosalina (*Melaleuca Ericifolia*)   This yellow essential oil is antiseptic and antibacterial. It's commonly used for muscle cramps. If you like rosewood, you'll also like rosalina. Rosalina is also known as lavender tea tree oil.

Rose, otto (*Rosa Damascena*)   This deep red essential oil is commonly used for fragrances, mature skin, dry skin, depression, menopause, and eczema. This is the queen of fragrances—and has the price tag to go along with it! It has a strong rose scent.

Rosemary (*Rosmarinus Officinalis*)   This green essential oil is analgesic, antimicrobial, and an antioxidant. It's commonly used for muscle cramps, dandruff, hair loss, arthritis, muscle aches, neuralgia, and rheumatism. The thick, greenish liquid of this plant is known as rosemary oleo resin. This can be added to oils to extend their shelf life. It has an herbal scent. *Do not use if you are pregnant, epileptic, or have high blood pressure.*

Rosewood (*Aniba Rosaedora*)   This light yellow essential oil is an antiseptic and a deodorant. It's commonly used for acne, scars, stretch marks, dry skin, colds, flu, fever, and headaches. It has a sweet woodsy and floral scent.

SAFETY FIRST

Rosewood is being overharvested. Consider using rosalina instead.

Sage, dalmatian (*Salvia Officinalis*)   This clear essential oil is anti-inflammatory, antibacterial, and antiseptic. Use it for oily skin, inflamed skin, acne, to stimulate hair growth, and to ease muscle pain. It has a harsh herbal fragrance. *Do not use if you are pregnant or have high blood pressure.*

Sage, Spanish (*Salvia Lavandulifolia*)   This clear essential oil is used for acne, dandruff, eczema, hair loss, dermatitis, rheumatism, coughing, headaches, asthma, colds, flu, and muscle cramps. It has all the therapeutic uses of *Salvia Officinalis*, without the dangers. *Do not use if you are pregnant.*

Sandalwood, mysore (*Santalum Album*)   This light yellow essential oil is an antiseptic, analgesic, and astringent. It's commonly used for colognes, eczema, aging skin, bronchitis, oily skin, scars, and stretch marks. It has a sweet woodsy scent.

Spearmint (*Mentha Spicata*)   This clear essential oil is used for headaches, vertigo, asthma, fever, and scabies. It's sweeter than peppermint but is less powerful, so it's good for children and the elderly. It has a minty scent.

Spikenard (*Nardostachys Jatamansi*)   This dark yellow essential oil is antifungal and is commonly used for dandruff, serious skin conditions, rashes, and wrinkles. It has a strong earthy scent.

Spruce (*Tsuga Canadensis*)   This clear essential oil is commonly used for muscle aches, pains, cramps, and depression. It has a woodsy scent.

Spruce, black (*Picea Mariana*)   This clear essential oil is used for muscle aches, pains, cramps, and depression. If you want that evergreen smell of the mountains, this is the one.

Styrax resin (*Liquidambar Styraciflua*)   This gold essential oil is antifungal and used to help with scabies. It smells similar to amber.

Tagetes (*Tagetes Glandulifera*)   This dark gold essential oil is antifungal. It's commonly used for warts and corns. *Do not use if you are pregnant. Do not use on small children. It is a sensitizer.*

Tangerine (*Citrus Reticulata*)   This green essential oil has antiseptic properties. It's used for muscle cramps, stretch marks, and acne, and also to clean hard surfaces. Tangerine is sweeter than mandarin. *It can be a sensitizer.*

Tansy, blue (*Tanacetum Anuum*)   This deep blue essential oil is anti-inflammatory, an antihistamine, and is nontoxic. It's commonly used for allergies, sunburns, damaged skin, respiratory problems, itching, bruises, nervous tension, muscle aches, sprains, and first aid. It has an herbal and lightly camphorous scent.

IN THE MIRROR

Blue tansy is not *Tanacetum Vulgare,* which aromatherapists warn against using. *Tanacetum Anuum* is mild and safe. You can use it in place of German chamomile or yarrow in skin care products. *Tanacetum Vulgare* is toxic.

Tea tree (*Melaleuca Alternifolia*)   This light yellow essential oil is antibiotic, antiseptic, antiviral, antibacterial, and antifungal. It's commonly used for repelling head lice and fleas, and for cold sores, colds, flu, ringworms, itching, insect bites, acne, pimples, headaches, sinusitis, sores, warts, and corns. It has a woodsy and herbal scent.

Tea tree, lemon-scented (*Leptospermum Petersonii*)   This light yellow essential oil has all the properties of tea tree, with the scent of lemon.

Thyme (*Thymus Vulgaris*)   This brown essential oil is antifungal, antiviral, and antibacterial. It's commonly used for muscle cramps, hair loss and dandruff, dermatitis, cuts, oily skin, insect bites, colds, and sore throat. It has an herbal scent.

Thyme, borneol (*Thymus Satureoides*) This reddish-brown essential oil is a great antimicrobial. It's commonly used in diffusers or room sprays for killing germs, bacteria, and viruses that are in the air. It's very strong and can be irritating to the skin, so it's not recommended for topical applications. Be sure to have this one in your arsenal to fight against germs when you have sick ones at home. It kills all the germs in a room when diffused or sprayed. It has an herbal scent.

Thyme, linalol (*Thymus Vulgaris Linalol*) This brown essential oil—the mildest of the thymes—is antibacterial, anti-infectious, and antifungal. It's commonly used for muscle cramps, hair loss and dandruff, dermatitis, cuts, oily skin, insect bites, colds, and sore throat. It has an herbal scent.

Vetiver, El Salvador (*Vetiveria Zizanoides*) This dark brown essential oil is commonly used for balancing sebum, men's cologne, oily skin, acne, sores, muscle aches, depression, rheumatism, and stress. It has a woodsy herbal and spicy scent.

Violet leaf (*Viola Odorata*) This dark green essential oil is an antiseptic. It's commonly used for soothing pain, aging skin, enlarged pores, blackheads, pimples, headaches, insomnia, bronchitis, sore throat, and stress. It has an earthy floral scent.

Yarrow (*Achillea Millefolium*) This dark blue essential oil has anti-inflammatory properties. It's commonly used for acne, oily skin, oily scalp, hair growth, painful muscles, wounds, headaches, fever, insomnia, varicose veins, scars, and stretch marks. It has a harsh woodsy and herbal scent. *Do not use if you are pregnant, or on babies or small children.*

Ylang ylang (*Canangium Odoratum*) This light yellow essential oil is commonly used for acne, balancing sebum, wrinkles, dermatitis, hair, sciatica, muscle spasms, insomnia, and exhaustion. It has a sweet floral and fruity fragrance.

The Least You Need to Know

- Be careful when measuring your essential oils, and be mindful of who they might be used on later. Some are very strong and can be a skin irritant.
- Blending certain essential oils together can be for more than just fragrance. They can have certain healing or soothing benefits.
- Along with their therapeutic properties, remember that essential oils are also useful for scenting your natural beauty products!

Helpful Herbs

In This Chapter

- What can herbs do for you?
- Infusing herbs
- Making extracts

Herbs have been in use for thousands of years. And not much has changed since those first people used them. We still use herbs for most of the same things early man did—as medicine, as disinfectants, to flavor foods, and to freshen the air. (They also used herbs for currency, but we've updated our money from leafy greens.)

You can use herbs in so many different products for a variety of illnesses and ailments, including acne, eczema, chapped feet and hands, dry skin, pain relief, dandruff, diaper rash, and many, many more! Some herbs get rid of pain, and fortunately, if they work for pain, they're usually antifungal, too—bonus!

You can use some herbs as is, but more often, you'll have to get the good stuff out of the herbs. To do this, you'll have to make extracts and infusions. You can then easily add the properties of the herb to your products or formulations.

Herbs for Making Beauty Products

Thinking about using *herbs* for hair care? Try aloe vera, arnica, birch, burdock, catmint, chamomile, horsetail, licorice, marigold, nettles, parsley, rosemary, sage, southernwood, or stinging nettle.

Some herbs help with pain, including angelica, arnica, ashok, ashwagandha, barberry, black cohosh, calendula, cayenne, cedar, celandine, chamomile, chaparral, comfrey root, feverfew, ginger, hops, kava kava, lavender, marshmallow, meadowsweet, motherwort, mullein, passion flower, poppy, reishi, skullcap, St. John's wort, turmeric, valerian, wild yam, and willow bark.

But that's just the tip of the iceberg! Let's look at all the herbs you can use when making your natural beauty products.

Açai (assai) berry (*Euterpe Oleracea*)   The açai berry contains vitamins B_1, B_2, B_3, C, and E; minerals; amino acids; and omega-6 and -9 fatty acids. It's anti-aging, anti-bacterial, and anti-inflammatory. It helps cell regeneration, pimples, acne, eczema, psoriasis, dry skin, mature skin, and damaged hair. Try it in creams, lotions, salves, balms, eye creams, lip products, and hair care products.

Açai has been found to be a very strong antioxidant and to contain vitamins that are supposed to regenerate the skin. It's also said to protect the collagen in our skin. Use infused açai in facial creams and lotions. Açai is also considered very good to use in creams for people with eczema and psoriasis.

Acerola berry (*Maldighia Glabra*)   The acerola berry contains vitamin C, iron, and calcium and is an antioxidant. It helps with dry skin and aids in fading age spots. Try it in lotions, creams, salves, and balms.

Alfalfa (*Medicago Sativa*) leaf   Alfalfa leaf helps with dry and itchy skin. Try it in facial cleansers, astringents, conditioners, eye creams, lotions, and toners. The ground seed is also used in bathwater to help relieve itchy skin. *Do not use if you are pregnant.*

Allspice (*Pimenta Dioica*)   Allspice is analgesic, anesthetic, antioxidant, antibacterial, antifungal, antiseptic, antiviral, and a muscle relaxer. It's commonly used in perfumes, soaps, and after-shaves. Try it in salves, lotions, and balms.

Aloe vera (*Aloe Barbadensis Miller*)   Aloe vera contains vitamins A, B_1, B_2, B_{12}, C, and E. It helps with rashes and sunburns, soothes skin, and promotes healing. It's commonly used in lotions, balms, salves, facials, masks, shaving creams, and facial creams. I often use aloe vera juice in place of, or in part for, water in creams, lotions, after-shave products, and baby products. Because it's so soothing, it's very good to use in creams and lotions for eczema and psoriasis.

Amla gooseberry; emblic myrobalan; Indian gooseberry (*Emblica Officinalis Gaertn, Phyllanthus Emblica*)   Amla is used to thicken and darken hair, to strengthen the hair strands, and for hair loss and alopecia, so try it in hair care products. This berry is being tested for use with treating bone disorders, diabetes, and HIV.

Arnica flowers (*Arnica Montana*)   The Native Americans used this wonderful herb extensively for pain relief. Today we can infuse it in oil and use it in salves for pain. When it's applied, you won't feel heat or cold like you do with commercial pain creams. Instead, after a little while, you'll simply realize you're no longer hurting. Triple-infuse this herb so it's very strong when you add it to your salves.

> **IN THE MIRROR**
>
> There was a time when those who used herbs to heal were put to death. Herbs were thought to be a form of witchcraft.

Arrowroot powder (*Maranta Arundinacea*)   Arrowroot has deodorizing, healing, and antibacterial properties. Use it for after-bath body powders, pimples, rashes, and wounds, and to absorb moisture. The feel of this powder is very smooth, and it softens the skin. In cosmetics, arrowroot can be used in place of talc, cornstarch, tapioca starch, potato starch, rice starch, or flour. It's excellent for use on dry, irritated, or sensitive skin.

Barley grass (*Hordeum Vulgare*)   Barley grass is an antioxidant. It contains vitamins A, B_1, B_2, B_{12}, and C; folic acid; calcium; iron; and potassium. Try it in hair care products, skin care products, and facials. It's good for all skin types.

Basil, holy; sacred basil (*Ocimum Sanctum*)   Basil has anti-aging properties. It's commonly used to strengthen hair and restore hair's manageability. Try it in facial creams, lotions, balms, hair care products, and salves.

Calendula (pot marigold) (*Calendula Officinalis*)   Calendula is an antifungal. It helps with dry or irritated skin, diaper rash, eczema, psoriasis, boils, and sores. Try it in lotions, balms, creams, hair conditioners, soaps, salves, after-bath powders, bath teas, and herb pillows. Calendula is known for its skin-soothing properties and is often used in soaps and many bath and body products. Infuse it in oil.

Chamomile (*Matricaria Chamomilla*)   Chamomile is antibacterial, antispasmodic, and healing. It helps heal rashes, abrasions, diaper rash, and burns. Use it for a calming tea, or in lotions, creams, salves, after-bath powders, bath teas, soaps, and baby products. Chamomile is wonderful for irritated skin. Infuse it in oil.

Cucumber; cucumber seeds (*Cucumis Sativus*)   Cucumber helps with dry and irritated skin and rashes. Try it in facial washes, toners, and soaps. Cucumber has a soothing effect on the skin, and it improves moisture retention.

Eclipta, bhringaraj; trailing eclipta (*Eclipta Alba*)   Eclipta helps with hair growth, covers graying, and darkens hair. You can make hair oil by boiling eclipta leaf juice in fractionated coconut oil.

Eucalyptus, blue gum (*Eucalyptus Globulus Labill*)   Eucalyptus is antiseptic, antiviral, antifungal, and antibacterial. It helps with insect bites, blisters, skin infections, cuts and wounds, herpes, and burns. Try it in candles to kill germs in the air and in salves, lotions, and after-shaves. The leaves can be used in room fresheners.

Fennel seeds; fennel roots (*Pimpinella Anisum*)   Fennel seed helps with the appearance of aging skin. It's also used in toothpastes, mouthwash, and soap.

Ginger; dried ginger (*Zingiber Officinale*)   Ginger is a stimulant, an anti-irritant, and an analgesic. It helps with joint and muscle pain. Try it in fragrances, after-shaves, soaps, teas, salves, balms, and bath oils. Both the dried herb and the essential oil are very fragrant and are often used as a scent.

Gotu kola (*Centella Asiatica*)   Gotu kola has healing properties and helps with shrinking and fading stretch marks. Try it in salves, creams, and lotions.

Henna; Cypress shrub; mehndi (*Lawsonia Inermis, Lawsonia Alba*)   Henna is used as a hair colorant, as a hair thickener, to add shine to hair, and for temporary tattoos. Henna is the only natural hair colorant approved by the Food and Drug Administration.

Hibiscus; hibiscus flower; red hibiscus; rose of China (*Hibiscus Rosa-Sinensis*) Hibiscus promotes hair growth; thickens hair; and is used in shampoos, conditioners, and rinses. It helps prevent premature graying and scalp disorders and is a dye for eyelashes and eyebrows.

Jasmine; jasmine flower; catalonian jasmine (*Jasminum Officinale, Jasminum Grandiflorum*) extracted oil   Jasmine helps with dry or irritated skin, mouth ulcers, and corns. It can be used in perfumes and cosmetics as well as in tinctures.

Karanja (*Pongamia Glabra*)   Karanja is a pesticide and is antiviral, antifungal, and antibacterial. It helps with eczema and psoriasis, and eases pain. It's safe for humans and pets. Try it in soaps, shampoos, lotions, and salves. For a head lice problem, use karanja added to regular store-bought shampoo to wash a child's hair. This is a safe way to remove the head lice and not expose the child to the pesticides in commercial head lice products.

Licorice (liquorice) (*Glycyrrhiza Glabra*)   Licorice has anti-inflammatory, astringent, and antimicrobial properties. It helps with eczema, herpes, shingles, sunburns, insect bites, light skin discolorations (absorbing UV rays), inflammations, burns, wounds, abscesses, boils, and other skin problems. Try it in lotions, creams, balms, and salves. *Do not use if you are pregnant or nursing.*

Mint; peppermint (*Mentha Piperita*)   Mint helps soothe aching feet and provides a refreshing feeling. Try it in lip products, creams, lotions, pain salves, shampoos, room sprays, balms, and soaps. Mint not only has a nice, clean, natural fragrance but also has other beneficial uses. Mint grows in several different varieties, and each has its own distinct scent.

SAFETY FIRST

Be very careful not to overuse peppermint. If you use too much in your product, it can burn sensitive skin and other tender areas. Diabetics should not use peppermint.

Myrrh; frankincense myrrh; mukul myrrh (*Commiphora Myrrha*)   Myrrh helps with pain relief, athlete's foot, infected wounds, skin inflammations, and irritated skin. Try it in tooth powders and gargles as well. Myrrh is like a little magic powder. You can relieve a painful sore throat by gargling with a small amount of myrrh dissolved in warm water. Add myrrh to your homemade tooth powder if you have cavities or gum disease. It's especially good for eczema. Use myrrh in talc for athlete's foot. It soothes irritated skin and is ideal in creams and lotions.

Nagarmotha (nutgrass) (*Cyperus Rotundus*)   Nagarmotha is an astringent and anti-inflammatory. It helps lighten the skin and is good to use in creams and lotions.

Neem tree; margosa tree parts (*Azadirachta Indica*)   Neem is antibacterial, antiviral, and antifungal. It helps with skin problems, acne, eczema, psoriasis, and sores and repels insects on pets. Try it in creams, lotions, soaps, shampoos, salves, and balms.

Use neem cakes around your house and in your garden to repel insects. You can also spray your trees, plants, and shrubs with a mixture of water and neem oil.

> **IN THE MIRROR**
>
> All parts of the neem tree are good to use for illnesses. In fact, the neem tree has been suggested to help with more than 40 different diseases.

Nettle leaves; nettle roots (*Urtica Dioica L*)   Nettle leaves help with stimulating hair growth, dandruff, dry hair, alopecia, and muscle and joint pain. It's a skin astringent, too. Try it in lotions, salves, and hair care products.

Oat (*Avena Sativa*)   Oat helps with dry skin, relives the itching of chicken pox, and exfoliates. Try it in creams, lotions, and shampoos.

Patchouli oil; patchouli seeds (*Pogostemon Cablin*)   Patchouli helps with chapped skin, razor bumps, and skin inflammation. Try it in perfumes, cosmetics, aftershaves, shaving lotions and creams, and soaps.

Rosemary (*Rosmarinus Officinalis*)   Rosemary is commonly used for lightening blond hair, conditioning, stimulating hair regrowth, and helping with alopecia. Try it in soaps, shampoos, lotions, creams, perfumes, and conditioners.

Spurge (*Euphorbia Hirta*)   Spurge helps with eczema, psoriasis, cracked lips, cracked hands, and cracked feet. Try it in lotions, creams, salves, and balms.

Sweet violet; viola (*Viola Odorata*)   Sweet violet helps with dry and itchy skin, eczema, oily skin, boils, insect bites, and snake bites, and it improves skin tone. Use it in creams, lotions, after-shave splashes, and facial toners. You can use this herb fresh or dry in tea bags or muslin bags in your bathwater to help with dry and itching skin.

Tea tree oil; tea tree leaves (*Melaleuca Alternifolia*)   Tea tree oil helps with skin cleansing, acne, athlete's foot, dandruff, hair care, and oral hygiene, and it repels lice. Try it in hair conditioners, lotions, creams, after-shave splashes, soaps, talcs, tinctures, and shampoos. It's recommended for external use only.

Tulsi (*Ocimum Sanctum*)   Tulsi is antibacterial. It can be used to lighten dark spots, and help with athlete's feet, sores, and ringworm. Try it in lotions, creams, talcs, hair conditioners, shampoos, and soaps.

Turmeric (*Curcuma Longa*)   Turmeric is antibacterial and antimicrobial. It helps with minor cuts and scrapes, eczema, and ringworm. Try it in creams and lotions.

Walnut; Persian walnut; European walnut (*Juglans Regia*)   Walnut helps eczema, itchy scalp, herpes, sunburns, acne, and dandruff. It helps exfoliate dry skin and is great in soaps and scrubs. Try it in salves and balms, too.

Extracts and Infusions

As mentioned at the start of this chapter, to get the benefits from herbs, you have to extract the goodness from them. You can then easily add the herbs' valuable qualities to lotions, bath potions, and other beauty products you make.

> **PRETTY POINTER**
>
> Remember to label and date each jar, whether it's an extract, infusion, or whatever. It's too easy to forget what's in that jar you just found pushed to the back of the cabinet!

Making Extracts

Extracts, also called tinctures, are made with alcohol, such as 100-proof vodka. The standard ratio when working with dry herbs is 1 part dried herb to 8 parts alcohol. Here's how it comes together:

1. In a coffee grinder, grind the herb until it's a powder.

2. Fill a sterile glass jar 1 inch full with the herb powder.

3. Fill the rest of the jar with alcohol. Cap the jar tightly, and shake.

4. Label the jar with the contents and the date. Store in a warm, dark place, out of direct light, for 2 weeks.

5. Strain the alcohol several times until all the pieces of the herb have been removed.

6. Bottle in a sterile bottle with a cap or fine mist sprayer.

Making Infusions

We often use infused oils in our lotions, creams, balms, and soaps. Infusing herbs into oil isn't difficult. However, straining the oil can be messy. Be sure to have plenty of paper towels handy before you start. I use coffee filters for the final straining. After your oil has been strained, you'll be able to see that the oil is a slightly different color.

Here's how to make infusions using the summer method:

1. Fill a sanitized glass canning jar half full with a dried herb, and fill the rest of the way with oil. I like to use high oleic sunflower oil or meadowfoam seed oil.

2. Add 1 teaspoon (4.9 milliliters) vinegar per 1 cup (236.6 milliliters) oil. Cap the jar tightly, and shake.

3. Label the jar with the contents and the date. Place in a sunny window or outside in the sun. Some say to leave 2 weeks; others say 6 weeks.

4. Strain the oil several times until all the pieces of the herb have been removed.

5. Replace the cap, and store in a cool, dark place until ready to use.

The vinegar extracts properties of the herb the oil can't. For a stronger extract, strain out the old herb, replace with new, and let it steep for another 2 to 6 weeks.

To make an infusion with the winter method:

1. Fill a canning jar half full with a dried herb, and fill the rest of the way with oil. Cap it tightly.

2. Place the jar in an ovenproof pan filled with enough water to come halfway up the side of the jar.

3. Place the pan in an oven set to the lowest setting. Leave for 8 hours.

4. Strain the oil several times until all the little pieces of the herb have been removed.

5. Replace the cap, and store in a cool, dark place until ready to use.

The Least You Need to Know

- Herbs have been used for healing since the ancient days; let's get back to using these wonderful gifts of nature!

- Herbs aren't just for seasoning your food! They also can help heal your skin and your hair.

- To use herbs, you have to get the good parts out of them. Extracts and infusions help you do that.

Pampering Skin and Body Products

In Part 2, we dive right into the beauty product recipes (and there are nearly 250 of them!), starting with clay and peel-off masks; lotions; creams; and all sorts of bath and body products like delicious body butters, bath oils, bombs, scrubs, and more.

Who needs a spa when you can create wonderful pampering products to use in your own home? And once you find out how easy and inexpensive it is to make your own bath and body products, you'll never want to use high-priced commercial products again. And the best part of all? Our recipes help you make all-natural and earth-friendly products.

Clays and Masks

In This Chapter

- Different kinds of clays
- The benefits of clays
- Matching a clay to your skin type
- Recipes for clay masks and facial peels

Is there anything more soothing and relaxing than a facial? Besides all the benefits facials give your skin, the time you spend relaxing during the facial gives you a chance to unwind, and when you're finished, you often have a fresh, rejuvenated look—and *outlook!*

All that comes from one simple concoction of clays and a few other ingredients. And in this chapter, we show you how to put them together.

The Importance of Labeling

For an anytime facial, you can keep small containers of your favorite clays or masks waiting for that special "me" time. Be sure to label your concoctions, though. What you may think is in the container or baggie may not actually be that. Add the date to the label as well. Time has a way of quickly flying by, and it's easy to forget just exactly what's in the containers and how long it's been there!

From time to time on one of the Yahoo! soap-making groups I'm part of, a member posts a funny story about something that happened to them while making soaps. Most of the other members can relate; funny things happen to us all when we're concocting. In fact, I've posted about several mishaps myself. So it's with a big smile that I share the following story. This is a true story, remember. I've added it with the author's permission. It will also remind you why it's so important to label things!

"I often mix up a batch of clay mask material into a container so that when I want a mask I just scoop a little out of it and add my liquid ingredients. It's been in that exact same container each and every time.

"A few weekends back I was letting my kids make M&P [melt-and-pour] soaps for fun and we made up some gnarly concoction of powders to add to glycerin for scenting and coloring some of the soaps.

"So last Friday afternoon, I felt like I could use a facial pick-me-up. So I was going to make myself a mask. I mixed it all up and applied it to my face. As I was doing so, I noticed it smelled horrid. It was downright gross-smelling, but I figured that could just be the sea kelp mixing with the lemon juice funny. (Lemon juice was handy so I chose to use that.) I went about my business trying to keep my dogs calm and make them stop barking at me because mommy looked so scary.

"After about an hour I was a little concerned that it had not yet hardened like the clay usually does. I touched a small part by my chin, and as I wiped it off from my chin I noticed that my face was not looking right. It had a funny color to it. So I wiped a little more off to see, and sure enough it was not my eyes tricking me, it was colored funny.

"Suddenly it hit me, as I begin laughing, crying, and screeching hysterically. I did not apply my clay mask mixture. What I had applied was the powder mix I made for my kids to tint their soaps. This mixture consisted of cocoa powder, rhassoul, kaolin clay, sea kelp powder, ground coffee, and best of all *henna* powder! Yes, *henna* powder. The kind of henna powder you mix with lemon juice to make henna tattoos! Frantically washing the monstrous mixture off my face, laughing and crying, I rinsed it off and looked in the mirror. Anyone who works with henna tattoos probably cringed at the adding lemon juice part, because lemon juice is an activator for the dye release in henna.

"I had two things going for me that would make it possible that I would not be wearing a tattoo on my entire face and neck for the next 2 to 6 weeks: I washed it off after an hour, and I did not put anything on that would normally enhance the staying power. By the end of the day, I had managed to scrub my face raw, while diminishing *some* of the harsh lines, but my eyebrows and hairline were a sight to be remembered!"

Clays and Their Benefits

Clays are used in facial products because of their ability to draw out toxins, impurities, and bacteria from the skin. Many draw out excess oils, which makes them great for people with oily skin or who have problems with acne. Clays are also used for their ability to tone, tighten, and exfoliate the skin.

Clays come in many colors, and you can even use them as natural colorants for soaps and lotions.

Certain clays are used as an important ingredient in foot and after-bath powders as well as in cosmetics. These clays come from volcanic ash.

There are three main groups of clays:

- Montmorillonite clays

- Illite clays

- Kaolinite clays

Montmorillonite clays have strong drawing properties and are exceptional for removing oils, toxins, and impurities from the skin. These are part of the smectite group, which means they absorb. They clear and cleanse the pores and help clear acne.

Illite clays get their coloring from the natural clay micas. Illites are not part of the smectite group. These clays are light and fluffy compared to the other clay groups. Certain clays in the illite group are said to be antibacterial; green illite clay is one of them. This group is used to cleanse and gently exfoliate the skin.

Kaolinite clays are used to stimulate blood circulation, exfoliate, and cleanse and nourish the skin. The kaolinite group is not part of the smectite group. These clays are widely used in cosmetics and many personal care products as well as in industrial manufacturing.

IN THE MIRROR

Many of these clay groups are used in treatment for medical problems both externally and internally—for example, detoxifying the body by absorbing the toxins from within. They can be used externally for pain relief or to protect and heal scrapes and cuts. You can even find some of these clays in your prescription medicines.

Bentonite Clay (Montmorillonite and Smectite Groups)

Bentonite is a light gray clay best used for oily skin. It draws out oils and toxins and exfoliates the skin. Many soap-makers add bentonite clay to their shaving soaps for the extra slip the razor needs for gliding while shaving. This clay is made of volcanic ash.

Do not use bentonite in a facial more than twice a week because it can draw out too much oil, leaving your skin dry.

French Green Clay (Montmorillonite and Smectite Groups)

French green clay is the favorite clay for use in cosmetics and spa treatments. It's very beneficial for skin problems such as acne. This clay draws out oils, toxins, and impurities from the skin while it also tightens pores. French green clay replenishes minerals and nutrients the skin needs to remain healthy.

Do not use this clay on sensitive or dry skin.

Green Illite Clay (Illite Group)

This green clay is different from the French green clay. This green clay is part of the illite group, which means it contains natural clay micas. It's light and fluffy with a pale green color. It gently removes dead skin and is the very best clay for drawing out toxins.

Because green illite clay draws out the oils, this clay is not recommended for those who have normal to dry skin.

Fuller's Earth (Montmorillonite and Smectite Groups)

Used for oily skin and for acne, fuller's earth has great oil-, toxin-, and bacteria-drawing properties and works wonders clearing and cleaning the pores.

This is the best clay to use for acne, but it's very drying, so don't use it more than once a week.

White Kaolin Clay (Kaolinite Group)

White kaolin or China clay is used in mineral makeup foundations, fillers, and blushes. This clay is light and very mild, and it does not absorb or draw oils. In facial masks, it's used for its gentle exfoliating, its ability to remove toxins, and its cleansing of the skin and pores.

This clay is the best choice for those with sensitive skin.

Pink, Red, Black, and Yellow Kaolin Clay (Kaolinite Group)

All these clays have the same characteristics as the white kaolin clay. They gently remove dead skin cells and toxins and restore and nourish the skin. The clays get their colors from clay micas. They're often used as natural colorants in soap-making.

These clays are all very mild and great for sensitive skin.

Moroccan Red Clay (Montmorillonite and Smectite Groups)

Best used for oily skin, Moroccan red clay removes dead skin, toxins, and bacteria; cleans pores; and tightens the skin. It is also used as a natural brick red colorant in soap-making.

It is, however, very drying and should not be used in a facial mask more than once a week. Those with sensitive skin should not use this clay.

Moroccan Rhassoul Clay (Montmorillonite and Smectite Groups)

This is a wonderful clay for all skin types and is used in spa body wraps as well as in facial masks. Rhassoul is rich in minerals and trace elements that nourish the skin while it removes the dead skin cells, toxins, bacteria, and impurities. The clay has a reddish-brown color.

Moroccan rhassoul is good for all skin types.

IN THE MIRROR

Ancient Egyptians and Romans used Moroccan rhassoul clay in cosmetics and as a medicine.

Rose Clay (Blend)

This clay is a blend made by mixing together equal parts French red illite and white kaolin clay. It's a very light and gentle clay used in cosmetics, facial masks, and as a natural colorant.

Use this clay on sensitive or dry skin.

Which Clay Is Best for Your Skin Type?

For the best results, it's important to match the clay to your skin type. This should help you tweak our recipes and make them more your own to fit your needs or wants.

For oily skin, try bentonite, French green, red kaolin, montmorillonite (blue and red), Moroccan red, or fuller's earth.

For normal skin, try Moroccan rhassoul, all the kaolinite clays, or green illite.

Making Facial Masks

Now for the fun stuff—time to make a mask! Creating your own facial masks isn't difficult, but I do recommend you follow a method for mixing the dry ingredients. First, you'll want to weigh all the dry ingredients according to the recipe and mix them together well. To do this, you'll need a scale. (We don't measure in volume using teaspoons, tablespoons, or cups, but actually weigh the ingredients using ounces.) Store the mask mixture in an airtight container—and be sure you label and date it! When you're ready to make a mask, remove the amount you need, add the liquid as specified in the recipe, stir until the mixture is spreadable, and apply. Easy!

Do try to set aside a little time each week for your "me" time and give yourself a wonderful facial. Soon you'll notice your skin looking younger, healthier, and more vibrant.

You may be wondering where you can find these clays, essential oils, and hydrosols. We have a list of online vendors in the back of the book. These are vendors we personally know, trust, and use ourselves.

IN THE MIRROR

One note before we begin: you'll notice in this and subsequent chapters, we don't include the amount of preservative or scent as part of the 100 percent makeup of these recipes. Scent is optional, and the amount of preservative depends on the type and brand of preservative you use. (See Appendix E for more on preservatives.)

Here's what you need to make facial masks:

- Scale
- Small plastic or glass container with a lid
- Spoon

Simple Milk and Clay Mask

We've always heard how beneficial milk is to the skin. This gentle and simple mask nourishes and cleanses your skin and is good for all skin types and ages. This recipe makes 4 ounces (113.6 grams) dry mix, or about 12 facials.

Clay (your choice)	2 ounces (56.7 grams)
Powdered milk	2 ounces (56.7 grams)

1. Using a food scale, put a bowl on the scale and push the tare button to zero out the weight of the bowl.

2. Weigh the dry ingredients one at a time, and place them in a bowl or small food grinder. We like to use a small grinder.

3. Return the bowl to the scale. It should still show zero weight. If not, push the tare button again and wait for it to zero out the weight of the bowl again. Continue with the next dry ingredient.

4. When you've weighed all the dry ingredients, grind them in the grinder for several seconds or until they're well incorporated. If using a bowl, stir them until they're well blended together.

5. Store the mixture in a baggie or airtight container until you're ready to use it.

To use:

1. Remove about 2 teaspoons (9.9 milliliters) dry mask mixture and hold in your hand or a small bowl.

2. Add any essential oils that may be part of the recipe, and stir well.

3. Add a few drops distilled water, hydrosol, or oil, and mix well.

4. Spread the mask over your clean, damp face and neck, avoiding your eye area.

5. Relax for 15 to 20 minutes while the mask works its magic.

6. When the mask is completely dry, rinse your face and neck with warm water. Pat it dry with a clean towel, and follow with a toner and moisturizer.

Dry Skin Mask

This is a wonderful hydrating mask for dry and/or mature skin. It removes the dead skin cells and draws out toxins while the sea kelp or sea mud gives extra skin-loving minerals. This recipe makes 3 ounces (85 grams) dry mix, or about 10 facials.

White kaolin clay	1 ounce (28.4 grams)
Moroccan rhassoul clay	1 ounce (28.4 grams)
Sea kelp or sea mud (powder form)	1 ounce (28.4 grams)

Prepare as directed in the Simple Milk and Clay Mask recipe. When ready to use, add to the dry mixture and stir well:

Chamomile essential oil	2 drops
Rose geranium essential oil	2 drops
Lavender essential oil	2 drops

Normal Skin Mask

This mask exfoliates, cleanses, nourishes, and brightens skin. That's why it's one of my favorites! It's good for all ages with normal skin types. For a change every once in a while, replace the distilled water with a rose hydrosol. This recipe makes 6 ounces (170.1 grams) dry mix, or about 20 facials.

Rose clay	2 ounces (56.7 grams)
Moroccan rhassoul clay	2 ounces (56.7 grams)
Sea kelp or sea mud (powder form)	2 ounces (56.7 grams)

Prepare as directed in the Simple Milk and Clay Mask recipe.

Oily Skin Mask

This is a good mask for those with oily skin but who don't have acne. It draws out toxins and excess oils while tightening pores and toning the skin. This recipe makes 6 ounces (170.1 grams) dry mix, or around 20 facials.

Finely ground oatmeal	1 ounce (28.4 grams)
Fuller's earth	2 ounces (56.7 grams)
Kaolin clay	3 ounces (85 grams)

Prepare as directed in the Simple Milk and Clay Mask recipe. When ready to use, add to the dry mixture and stir well:

Clary sage essential oil	2 drops
Lemon essential oil	2 drops
Rosemary essential oil	2 drops

Oily Problem Skin Mask

This mask is great for acne suffers. It pulls out toxins, oils, and grime from deep in the pores. It's not recommended for use more than once or twice a week, though. This recipe makes 6 ounces (170.1 grams) dry mix, or about 20 masks.

Fuller's earth	2 ounces (56.7 grams)
Moroccan rhassoul clay	2 ounces (56.7 grams)
Finely ground oatmeal	2 ounces (56.7 grams)

Prepare as directed in the Simple Milk and Clay Mask recipe. When ready to use, add to the dry mixture and stir well:

Clary sage essential oil	1 drop
Juniper essential oil	1 drop
Rosemary essential oil	1 drop
Patchouli essential oil	1 drop
Ylang ylang essential oil	1 drop

IN THE MIRROR

Açai oil has been on the market for a while. It has wonderful benefits for internal and external use; however, it is very expensive. Recently a butter has become available that has a 25 percent açai berry content. The butter is a much more economical way to get the benefits of the açai berry without the high cost. Try it in dry or mature skin hydrating facials.

Delicious Chocolate and Strawberry Mask

The combination of cocoa powder and fruit powders in masks has become very popular. And with good reason! Cocoa powder contains many important antioxidants, and the fruit powders are packed with vitamins and help loosen dead skin cells. The honey and yogurt powder each bring their own benefits, too. This recipe makes about 5 masks.

Kaolin clay (your choice)	.5 ounce (14.2 grams)
Powdered milk	.5 ounce (14.2 grams)
Honey powder	.1 ounce (2.8 grams)
Cocoa powder	.5 ounce (14.2 grams)
Yogurt powder	.2 ounce (5.7 grams)
Strawberry powder	.2 ounce (5.7 grams)

Prepare as directed in the Simple Milk and Clay Mask recipe.

Rejuvenating Mask

The use of green tea powder and pomegranate powder gives this mask cell revital-izing and antioxidant properties. This recipe makes about 5 masks.

Kaolin clay (your choice)	1 ounce (28.4 grams)
Sea kelp or Dead Sea mud (powder form)	.5 ounce (14.2 grams)
Green tea powder	.3 ounce (8.5 grams)
Pomegranate powder	.2 ounce (5.7 grams)

Prepare as directed in the Simple Milk and Clay Mask recipe.

Making Facial Peels

Along with masks, the time you spend doing a facial peel is all your own time. You can lock yourself away and relax while your skin is being rejuvenated. Facial peels not only pull out black- and whiteheads from your pores; they also remove dead skin and dirt left behind after washing. For most people, the worst areas for blackheads are around the nose and chin, so that's the first place you'll want to apply your facial peel. And as with the clays, avoid getting the peel near your eyes.

When you're ready to remove the peel, start peeling the mask from your forehead down. Always rinse your face after a peel and follow it with a toner and moisturizer.

Here's what you need to make a facial peel:

- Stove
- Small saucepan
- Spoon
- Small bowl
- Refrigerator

Simple Facial Peel

This quick and easy peel is just what your skin needs for a little pick-me-up. This recipe makes 1 facial peel.

Distilled water	1 ounce (28.4 grams)
Unflavored gelatin	.25 ounce (7.1 grams)
Aloe vera gel or juice	1 ounce (28.4 grams)
Oil (your choice)	.1 ounce (2.8 grams)

1. In a small saucepan over medium heat, bring the distilled water to a boil and add the gelatin. Stir while the gelatin dissolves and then remove the pan from heat.

2. Add aloe vera gel and oil, and stir well.

3. Pour the mixture into a small bowl, and refrigerate for about 20 minutes or until the mixture becomes thick.

4. Spread the mixture over your clean, damp face and neck, avoiding your eye area. Relax while the peel dries.

5. Peel off the dried mask, starting at your forehead. Follow by rinsing your face with warm water.

PRETTY POINTER

If you don't want to use an animal by-product such as the gelatin, try replacing the unflavored gelatin called for in these recipes with .2 ounce (5.7 grams) xanthan gum. I've not tested this method, but I've heard it works. The directions would be the same as if you were using the unflavored gelatin.

Facial Peel for Mature Skin

This is a great one-time-use peel. This recipe makes 1 facial peel.

Distilled water	1.5 ounces (42.5 grams)
Unflavored gelatin	.25 ounce (7.1 grams)
Aloe vera juice	.5 ounce (14.2 grams)
White kaolin clay	.2 ounce (5.7 grams)
Sea kelp or mud (powder form)	.2 ounce (5.7 grams)
Iris florentina extract (anti-aging)	.1 ounce (2.8 grams)

Prepare as directed in the Simple Facial Peel recipe.

PRETTY POINTER

For extra skin-loving benefits, try steeping a few herbs in the distilled water. Strain the herbs from the water before you continue making your mask or peel.

Facial Peel for Oily Skin

This one-time-use peel is perfect for oily and acne-prone skin. Don't forget to smooth it on your neck, too! This recipe makes 1 facial peel.

Distilled water	1.5 ounces (42.5 grams)
Unflavored gelatin	.25 ounce (7.1 grams)
Aloe vera juice	.5 ounce (14.2 grams)
Rosemary essential oil	2 drops
Cypress or juniper berry essential oil	2 drops

Prepare as directed in the Simple Facial Peel recipe.

The Least You Need to Know

- Clay masks can improve your skin, no matter your skin type or age.
- Follow your skin type to determine what type of clay is best to use in your masks.
- Always label and date your containers.
- Remember to take some "me" time and relax while giving yourself a facial!

All Things Facial

In This Chapter

- Soothing facial creams and cleansers
- Excellent exfoliants
- Facial balms to soothe your skin
- Terrific facial toners

In this chapter, we've included lots of skin care product recipes, so you're sure to find some well suited for your skin type.

We hope you have a blast making these cleansers, exfoliants, and more, but be sure to *use* them! These products won't do much for your skin if they sit idle on your bathroom counter or nightstand, unused. (I know this because I'm terrible about remembering to use my products daily!) They do, however, work *wonders* when you actually use them!

The Basics of Making Facial Products

Cleansers, creams, and toners are an important part of taking care of your skin, especially your face. Having a daily regimen in place—and following it!—helps keep your skin healthy and youthful.

Here's what you need to make the goodies in this chapter:

- Stove
- Scale
- Several glass or plastic bowls
- 8-quart stockpot
- Spoons or whisk

- Funnel
- Thermometer (meat or candy type)
- Immersion blender
- Sanitized jars and bottles

IN THE MIRROR

As noted earlier, we don't include the amount of preservative or scent as part of the 100 percent makeup of these recipes. Scent is optional, and the amount of preservative depends on the type and brand of preservative you use. (See Appendix E.) I like Optiphen Plus preservative for these recipes. It's paraben- and formaldehyde-free.

Making Facial Creams

Facial creams are thick creams useful for very dry skin or for mature skin. During the winter, you can use these creams daily to help prevent your skin from drying out due to the cold weather.

Extreme Facial Crème

With the winter's cold, you'll find this cream very soothing. Even though this cream is very thick and heavy, it soaks in nicely, leaving your skin moisturized and protected from the cold. Those with very dry, mature skin may find this cream perfect for year-round moisturizing. This recipe makes 16 ounces (453.6 grams). You'll need 1 (16-ounce; 453.6-gram) jar, 2 (8-ounce; 226.8-gram) jars, or 4 (4-ounce; 113.4-gram) jars.

Evening primrose oil	2.5 ounces (70.9 grams)
Mango butter	1.5 ounces (42.5 grams)
Meadowfoam oil	1.5 ounces (42.5 grams)
Avocado oil	1.4 ounces (39.7 grams)
Pumpkin seed oil	1 ounce (28.4 grams)
Cocoa butter	.5 ounce (14.2 grams)
Emulsifying wax	1.2 ounces (34 grams)
Stearic acid	.5 ounce (14.2 grams)
Distilled water	6.1 ounces (172.9 grams)
Preservative	(see manufacturer's recommendation)
Skin-safe fragrance or essential oil	.2 ounces (5.7 grams)

1. Set your scale to ounces. Place a bowl on the scale, and push the tare button to zero out the weight of the bowl. Weigh your liquids one at a time in a bowl, and place them in a stockpot. Heat over low heat until the oils and butters completely melt.

2. Bring the oils and butters to a temperature of 180°F. If you're using unrefined butter, hold the mixture at that temperature for 20 minutes. This kills any germs or bacteria that may be in the unrefined butter.

3. Weigh the emulsifying wax and stearic acid, and add these to the pot.

4. While the wax is melting, weigh and warm the distilled water in a saucepan over medium heat. Your water has to be warm before you add it to the mixture; otherwise, the water will cool the oils and you won't get a good emulsion.

5. Add water to the mixture, and use an immersion blender to bring the mixture together to form a good emulsion. Remove the pot from the heat.

6. When the mixture has cooled to 110°F, add the preservative and fragrance. Use the immersion blender again to incorporate all the ingredients. At this time, you can also add a skin-safe colorant. Let the mixture completely cool.

As the mixture cools, it will thicken into a beautiful, rich cream. Package in sterile jars.

SAFETY FIRST

Be careful not to overheat your oils in step 2. Overheated butter, such as mango or cocoa butter, will crystallize later on and feel grainy in the finished product.

Açai Face Butter

This is a very rich, very thick, yet still light facial butter that contains all the benefits of the açai berry. Açai is well known for its anti-aging properties. This recipe is perfect for mature skin, for those who spend a lot of time in the sun, and for those who want to prevent premature wrinkles. This recipe makes 24 ounces (680.4 grams).

Açai-infused sunflower oil	3 ounces (85 grams)
Shea butter (cosmetic grade)	3 ounces (85 grams)
Evening primrose oil	2 ounces (56.7 grams)
Avocado oil	2 ounces (56.7 grams)
Pumpkin seed oil	1 ounce (28.4 grams)
Cocoa butter	.7 ounce (19.8 grams)
Emulsifying wax	1.9 ounces (53.9 grams)
Stearic acid	.7 ounce (19.8 grams)
Vegetable glycerin	.7 ounce (19.8 grams)
DL panthenol B_5 (vitamin B_5)	.25 ounce (7.1 grams)

Distilled water	9 ounces (225.1 grams)
Fragrance or essential oil	.25 ounce (7.1 grams)
Preservative	(see manufacturer's recommendation)

Prepare as directed in the Extreme Facial Crème recipe, and package in sterile jars.

> **PRETTY POINTER**
>
> Açai berries are packed full of skin- and cell-saving benefits. To create the açai–sunflower oil infusion, see Chapter 4. When using crushed berries, fill a 1-quart (32-ounce; 907.2-gram) canning jar half full of the crushed berries and add 8 ounces (226.8 grams) oil. (No need to weigh the berries.) If the berries are very powdery, fill the jar 1 inch (2.54 centimeters) full with the powder and follow with 8 ounces (226.8 grams) oil.

Light Facial Cream

This cream, formulated for those who need a little more than a lotion, isn't as heavy as the other creams, so it's suitable for younger dry skin or normal mature skin. This recipe makes 16 ounces (453.6 grams). Use 2 (8-ounce; 226.8-gram) jars.

Sweet almond oil	2 ounces (56.7 grams)
Evening primrose oil	1.7 ounces (48.2 grams)
Macadamia nut oil	1 ounce (28.4 grams)
Emulsifying wax	1.3 ounces (36.9 grams)
Distilled water	10 ounces (283.5 grams)
Fragrance or essential oil	.2 ounce (5.7 grams)
Preservative	(see manufacturer's recommendation)

Prepare as directed in the Extreme Facial Crème recipe, and package in sterile jars.

Anti-Aging Facial Cream for Younger Skin

So you're 30-something and beginning to notice a few tiny fine lines near your eyes or around your mouth. This cream will help hold those fine lines at bay. Don't panic that this recipe has several specialty ingredients. They come from Lotion Crafter, an online supply business (see Appendix D). The meadowfoam seed oil pulls the anti-aging ingredients deep into the tissues. This recipe makes 16 ounces (453.6 grams).

You can halve this recipe to make only 8 ounces (226.8 grams) or even double it, if desired.

Shea butter	3.2 ounces (90.7 grams)
Meadowfoam seed oil	2.4 ounces (68 grams)
Emulsifying wax	1 ounce (28.4 grams)
Aloe vera juice or distilled water	8.3 ounces (235.3 grams)
Fragrance or essential oil	.2 ounce (5.7 grams)
Preservative	(see manufacturer's recommendation)

After the mixture has cooled to under 104°F, add:

Arireline (for wrinkles)	.5 ounce (14.2 grams)
Coenzyme Q-10 (anti-aging)	.3 ounce (8.5 grams)

Prepare as directed in the Extreme Facial Crème recipe, and package in sterile jars.

PRETTY POINTER

You can always use distilled water in place of aloe vera juice. In recipes that call for half aloe vera and half distilled water, you can use 100 percent distilled water.

Anti-Aging Facial Cream for Mature Skin

I formulated this cream for myself, and I love it so much I wanted to share it with you. This recipe easily can be cut in half or doubled. If you want to tweak it a little, try swapping argan oil for the evening primrose oil. This recipe makes 8 ounces (226.8 grams).

Meadowfoam seed oil	.7 ounce (19.8 grams)
Pumpkin seed oil	.5 ounce (14.2 grams)
Evening primrose oil	.5 ounce (14.2 grams)
Emulsifying wax	.4 ounce (11.3 grams)
Aloe vera juice or distilled water	5.2 ounces (147.4 grams)

After the cream has cooled to 104°F, add:

Coenzyme Q-10-Q-Max	.24 ounce (6.8 grams)
Iris florentina extract	.16 ounce (4.5 grams)
Hyaluronic acid	.08 ounce (2.3 grams)

Prepare as directed in the Extreme Facial Crème recipe. When the cream has cooled to 104°F, add:

LC Wrinkle Defense	.24 ounce (6.8 grams)
Essential or fragrance oil	.08 ounce (2.3 grams)
Preservative	(see manufacturer's recommendation)

Package in sterile jars.

Anti-Aging Eye Cream

This cream is wonderful for helping minimize folds on the eyelid, wrinkles, and under-eye bags. You will see a definite difference after using for 4 weeks, but don't stop. Keep on using the cream to continue the effects! This recipe makes 4 ounces (113.4 grams).

Meadowfoam seed oil	.5 ounce (14.2 grams)
Evening primrose oil	.5 ounce (14.2 grams)
Emulsifying wax	.2 ounce (5.7 grams)
Aloe vera juice or distilled water	2.6 ounces (73.7 grams)

Prepare as directed in the Extreme Facial Crème recipe. When cream has cooled to 104°F, add:

Eyeseryl	.4 ounce (11.3 grams)
LC Wrinkle Defense	.1 ounce (2.8 grams)
Preservative	(see manufacturer's recommendation)

Package in a sterile 4-ounce (113.4-gram) jar.

Moisturizing Facial Cream

This lotion is suitable for those who have slightly dry skin. It's light enough to put under makeup but heavy enough to keep your skin well moisturized all day. This is my moisturizer of choice under my makeup. This recipe can be cut in half or even doubled. Either way will work just fine. This recipe makes 32 ounces (907.2 grams).

Avocado oil	1.8 ounces (51 grams)
Peach kernel oil	1.4 ounces (39.7 grams)
Meadowfoam seed oil	1.4 ounces (39.7 grams)

Castor oil	1.4 ounces (39.7 grams)
Emulsifying wax	2.6 ounces (73.7 grams)
Stearic acid	.4 ounce (11.3 grams)
Distilled water	14 ounces (396.9 grams)
Aloe vera gel or juice	8.25 ounces (233.9 grams)
Fragrance or essential oil	.3 ounce (8.5 grams)
Preservative	(see manufacturer's recommendation)

Prepare as directed in the Extreme Facial Crème recipe, and package in sterile jars.

Light Moisturizer

This lotion is for those with normal skin who just need a light, under-makeup moisturizer. This recipe makes 24 ounces (680.4 grams).

Safflower oil	2.9 ounces (82.2 grams)
Avocado oil	2.9 ounces (82.2 grams)
Peach kernel oil	2.9 ounces (82.2 grams)
Sweet almond oil	2.9 ounces (82.2 grams)
Emulsifying wax	1.9 ounces (53.9 grams)
Aloe vera juice	10.6 ounces (300.5 grams)
Fragrance or essential oil	.25 ounce (7.1 grams)

Prepare as directed in the Extreme Facial Crème recipe, and package in sterile jars or bottles.

Making Facial Cleansers

Soap alone won't remove 100 percent of the makeup, grime, oil, and pollutants that collect on our faces every day. To get your face totally clean, you need a good cleansing cream. And you're in luck! We've included three in this section to help you get started making your own cleansing creams.

They're simple to use: after you've rubbed the cleanser over your face, just wipe it all off with a tissue. After using a cleanser, use a toner and then a moisturizer to make your skin glow.

Cold Cream

Cold creams have been around forever for removing makeup and moisturizing our skin. Here's a simple but good recipe I know you will enjoy. You can cut this recipe in half or double it if desired. This recipe makes 16 ounces (453.6 grams).

Beeswax	4 ounces (113.4 grams)
Sweet almond oil	4 ounces (113.4 grams)
Castor oil	4 ounces (113.4 grams)
Aloe vera juice	4 ounces (113.4 grams)
Fragrance or essential oil	1 teaspoon (4.9 milliliters)
Preservative	(see manufacturer's recommendation)

1. On the stove over medium-low heat, melt the weighed beeswax.

2. Add the oils and aloe vera juice to the wax, and stir well. Let the oils warm to 110°F and then remove from heat.

3. Add the fragrance oil and preservative, and mix well.

4. Pour into sterile jars and let completely cool. The mixture will thicken as it cools. Place lid on jars.

Sunflower Facial Cleansing Cream

This cleanser is best suited for dry or mature skin. This recipe makes 16 ounces (453.6 grams).

Sunflower oil	1 ounce (28.4 grams)
Apricot kernel oil	.7 ounce (19.8 grams)
Sweet almond oil	.7 ounce (19.8 grams)
Castor oil	.7 ounce (19.8 grams)
Emulsifying wax	.8 ounce (22.7 grams)
Stearic acid	.3 ounce (8.5 grams)
Distilled water	11.6 ounces (328.9 grams)
Fragrance or essential oil	.2 ounce (5.7 grams)
Preservative	(see manufacturer's recommendation)

Prepare as directed in the Cold Cream recipe.

Facial Cleansing Cream for Problem Skin

This recipe is for those who have acne and other types of problem skin. Jojoba oil doesn't aggravate acne because it's not an oil but a liquid wax. Jojoba oil moisturizes the skin and also cuts through makeup, pollution, and grime. This recipe makes 16 ounces (453.6 grams).

Jojoba oil	2.6 ounces (73.7 grams)
Distilled water	10 ounces (283.5 grams)
Aloe vera gel	2 ounces (56.7 grams)
Stearic acid	.3 ounce (8.5 grams)
Emulsifying wax	1.1 ounces (31.2 grams)
Lemongrass essential oil	.2 ounce (5.7 grams)
Preservative	(see manufacturer's recommendation)

Prepare as directed in the Cold Cream recipe.

Making Exfoliants

Exfoliants remove all the dead cells from your skin, leaving it soft and with a much more youthful glow and texture. It's important to exfoliate at least once a week to keep your skin looking its best. Even people who have problem skin still need to exfoliate, and we have the perfect recipe for you! Exfoliants aren't hard to make and pay back your efforts with refreshed and glowing skin.

Avena Facial Cleanser and Exfoliant

This quick but effective cleanser and exfoliant is so easy to whip up. It's ready to use as soon as you get it in the jar. This recipe makes 11.5 ounces (326 grams).

Moisturizing cream (your choice)	8 ounces (226.8 grams)
Finely ground oatmeal	¼ cup (59.2 milliliters)
Rosemary oleo resin	1 teaspoon (4.9 milliliters)
Rose geranium essential oil	.1 ounce (2.8 grams)
Preservative	(see manufacturer's recommendation)

1. Place a bowl on top of your scale, and push the tare button to zero out the weight of the bowl. Weigh your moisturizing cream and place in a medium bowl.

2. Replace the smaller bowl on the scale, and again push the tare button. Now weigh each ingredient one at a time and place them in the medium bowl.

3. Mix the ingredients together well and pour into a sterile jar.

IN THE MIRROR

Avena is another word for "oatmeal." You can use a coffee grinder to grind the oats.

Jojoba Exfoliant

This is an excellent exfoliant for people with problem skin or acne. Jojoba oil does not aggravate acne. This recipe is a cold mix, which means you just weigh and stir it all together. Easy as 1-2-3! This recipe makes 8 ounces (226.8 grams).

Jojoba oil	6 ounces (170.1 grams)
LipidThix	1.2 ounces (34 grams)
Jojoba beads	1 tablespoon (14.8 milliliters)
Bergamot essential oil	½ teaspoon (2.5 milliliters)
Rose geranium essential oil	½ teaspoon (2.5 milliliters)
Preservative	(see manufacturer's recommendation)

Prepare as directed in the Avena Facial Cleanser and Exfoliant recipe, and package in sterile jars.

IN THE MIRROR

LipidThix is a product we buy at Lotion Crafters. By adding it, you can make any oil thick, like an emulsion or a butter. For most oils, you use 20 percent LipidThix and 80 percent oil to make a thick butter that will support jojoba beads or ground kernel such as apricot—perfect for making a scrub or exfoliant!

Oatmeal Exfoliant

We all know how well oatmeal works as a gentle exfoliant, and this recipe takes advantage of that! It's so quick and easy, there's no heating involved. Just weigh all the ingredients, put in a jar, and it's ready to use. If you prefer, substitute brown sugar in place of the white. They both do the same thing for the skin. This recipe makes 2.5 ounces (70.9 grams).

Sweet almond oil	1 ounce (28.4 grams)
Finely ground oatmeal	.5 ounce (14.2 grams)
Fine white sugar	.5 ounce (14.2 grams)
Preservative	(see manufacturer's recommendation)

Prepare as directed in the Avena Facial Cleanser and Exfoliant recipe, and package in sterile jars.

PRETTY POINTER

Using sugar, either white or brown, in a scrub or exfoliant helps with problem skin or acne. The sugar "eats" the bacteria off the skin, helping clear up the complexion. Try tweaking your favorite recipe by adding an ounce or two of sugar.

Making Facial Balms

Facial balms are wonderful for protecting the skin if you're going to be outside in the weather. For those times you know you'll be out in the sun, you might want to add a little Z-Cote zinc oxide for UV protection, even in winter. (If you plan on using the balm at night, you can skip the zinc.)

Balms are made mainly of oil, butter, and wax. (Because of this, most of them feel pretty greasy when you first apply them. But never fear; they do sink into the skin nicely after a few minutes.) For the wax, you can choose to use only one or make a blend. Please don't use a petroleum-base wax. They are harmful to your skin and are not intended to be used on it. Instead, choose one or a combination of these:

- Beeswax
- Soy wax
- Candelilla
- Carnauba
- Another vegetable wax

Essential oils are great additives for these balms. Rather than choosing an essential oil for its scent, choose one whose properties target your skin needs.

Dry Skin Facial Balm

Even during the summer I use this facial balm. It's light and soaks quickly into the skin, but it still leaves a slightly slick feel so it's better to use at night and not during the day when you'll also be wearing makeup. This recipe makes 32 ounces (907.2 grams).

Lanolin	14.1 ounces (399.7 grams)
Shea butter	7 ounces (198.4 grams)
Glycerin	6 ounces (170.1 grams)
Hempseed oil	3.8 ounces (107.7 grams)
Vitamin E	.6 ounce (17 grams)
Z-Cote zinc oxide	.5 ounce (14.2 grams)
Bergamot essential oil	.25 ounce (7.1 grams)
Lavender essential oil	.25 ounce (7.1 grams)
Litsea essential oil	.15 ounce (4.3 grams)
Preservative	(see manufacturer's recommendation)

1. Weigh the wax and place it in a medium saucepan. Heat over medium-low heat until it's just about all melted.

2. Weigh the butters and add them to the saucepan. Reduce heat to low. When the butters have just about melted, remove the pan from the heat and stir to help the butters finish melting the rest of the way. (If you'd rather, you can microwave the wax and butters in a microwave-safe dish in 1 minute spurts, stirring in between, until they've just about melted. Stir while they finish melting.)

3. Weigh the oils, add them to the melted wax and butter, and stir well.

4. Let the balm cool to 110°F and then add the fragrance (if using) and preservative, and stir well.

5. While still hot, pour into sterile jars. Let completely cool and place the lids on the jars.

PRETTY POINTER

If you're allergic to lanolin or don't want to use it, substitute castor jelly instead. You might need to add a small amount of stearic acid for a little more firmness. Also, butters can become grainy or gritty if they get too hot while melting. To avoid this, use low heat and remove them from the heat source before all the butter has melted. Stir them while they finish melting.

Snow Ski Facial Balm

This is a perfect facial balm to protect the skin while you're out in the cold wind skiing or just playing. Z-Cote zinc oxide helps protect against UV rays as well, and doesn't leave a white coating on the skin. This recipe makes 8 ounces (226.8 grams).

Beeswax pastilles	2.6 ounces (73.7 grams)
Shea butter	1.3 ounces (36.9 grams)
Cocoa butter	1 ounce (28.4 grams)
Avocado oil	1.1 ounces (31.2 grams)
Sweet almond oil	1.2 ounces (34 grams)
Z-Cote zinc oxide	.6 ounce (17 grams)
Fragrance or essential oil	.2 ounce (5.7 grams)
Preservative	(see manufacturer's recommendation)

Prepare as directed in the Dry Skin Facial Balm recipe, and package in sterile jars.

IN THE MIRROR

Z-Cote zinc oxide won't leave a white film on your skin the way the old zinc oxide used to. It's completely clear when used in formulations.

Kokum Butter Moisturizing Facial Balm

This facial balm is full of skin-loving butters and oils to protect and soften the skin. Kokum butter may be a little hard to find, but it's worth the hunt. It adds much-needed vitamins as well as a protective seal to hold moisture in and everything else out, yet your skin can still breathe. You can cut this recipe down by halves or double it if you desire. This recipe makes 26 ounces (737.1 grams).

Soy wax or Joy Wax (We love Joy Wax.)	6 ounces (170.1 grams)
Shea butter	6 ounces (170.1 grams)
Kokum butter	4 ounces (113.4 grams)

Jojoba oil	4 ounces (113.4 grams)
Sesame oil	4 ounces (113.4 grams)
Squalane	2 ounces (56.7 grams)
Vitamin E	1 gel cap
Lavender essential oil	.35 ounce (9.9 grams)
Peppermint essential oil	.07 ounce (2 grams)
Preservative	(see manufacturer's recommendation)

Prepare as directed in the Dry Skin Facial Balm recipe, and package in deodorant push-up tubes.

Making Facial Toners

Facial toners work in two ways: they remove any leftover dirt or grime your soap or cleanser left behind, and they close your pores, keeping future dirt and grime out. That second item is an important step that shouldn't be overlooked or omitted from your daily cleansing.

Your skin type determines the type of toner you should use. Those with sensitive skin should stick with a toner that contains aloe vera but no alcohol. Those with acne need witch hazel and alcohol.

As you'll see, these toners are easy to make. Use a baby eye dropper to add the essential oils.

Facial Toner for Normal to Dry Skin

This light and gentle toner removes any remaining dirt and oil from your skin and closes your pores. And it's not too harsh for dry skin. This recipe makes 4 ounces (113.4 grams).

Rose water (We like Cortas brand.)	3.6 ounces (102.1 grams)
Polysorbate 20	.4 ounce (11.3 grams)
Palmarosa essential oil	4 drops
Geranium essential oil	4 drops
Preservative	(see manufacturer's recommendation)

1. In a sterile bottle, mix together all ingredients.

2. Alternatively, you can prepare a large batch and pour it into several sterile bottles.

Facial Toner for Normal to Sensitive Skin

This toner is gentle yet very effective. You'll love using the rose hydrosol! And yes, it does have a very light rose scent. This recipe makes 4 ounces (113.4 grams).

Aloe vera juice	1.4 ounces (39.7 grams)
Rose hydrosol	1 ounce (28.4 grams)
Glycerin	1 ounce (28.4 grams)
Polysorbate 20	.4 ounce (11.3 grams)
Lavender essential oil	4 drops
Ylang ylang essential oil	4 drops
Preservative	(see manufacturer's recommendation)

Prepare as directed in the Facial Toner for Normal to Dry Skin recipe.

Facial Toner for Rosacea

Rosacea can be very difficult to clear and keep clear. This toner has the healing of chamomile and green tea. You can use loose tea or tea bags to brew the teas. This recipe makes 4 ounces (113.4 grams).

Brewed green tea	1 ounce (28.4 grams)
Brewed chamomile tea	1 ounce (28.4 grams)
Witch hazel	1 ounce (28.4 grams)
Polysorbate 20	.4 ounce (11.3 grams)
Rose hip oil	.6 ounce (17 grams)
Preservative	(see manufacturer's recommendation)

1. Brew the teas using distilled water. You can use a normal amount of loose tea leaves as you would for a cup of tea to drink, or you can use 1 tea bag. Let steep a few minutes. Strain and then weigh 1 ounce (28.4 grams) of each green tea and chamomile tea.

2. Weigh and add the witch hazel, Polysorbate 20, and rose hip oil.

3. Let cool to less than 110°F and add preservative. Bottle.

Facial Toner for Oily Skin

Oily skin needs extra care to prevent breakouts. The essential oil blend in this recipe is designed to help control the oil, close the pores, and control the bacteria that adhere to the skin due to the oil. You may halve or double this recipe if desired. This recipe makes 4 ounces (113.4 grams).

Witch hazel	3.6 ounces (102.1 grams)
Polysorbate 20	.4 ounces (11.3 grams)
Eucalyptus essential oil	4 drops
Peppermint essential oil	2 drops
Rosemary essential oil	2 drops.
Preservative	(see manufacturer's recommendation)

Prepare as directed in the Facial Toner for Normal to Dry Skin recipe.

Facial Toner for Acne

After you've exfoliated, you'll need to follow with this toner, which closes those pores and helps prevent future breakouts. This recipe makes 4 ounces (113.4 grams).

Witch hazel	2.6 ounces (73.7 grams)
Aloe vera gel	1 ounce (28.4 grams)
Polysorbate 20	.4 ounce (11.3 grams)
Lavender essential oil	4 drops
Rosemary essential oil	4 drops
Lemongrass essential oil	4 drops
Preservative	(see manufacturer's recommendation)

Prepare as directed in the Facial Toner for Normal to Dry Skin recipe.

Rose Water Facial Toner

For mature skin, there's nothing as soothing and beneficial as a rose water toner. You'll love the light rose fragrance, too! This recipe makes 8 ounces (226.8 grams).

Rose water (We like Cortas brand.)	2 ounces (56.7 grams)
Lavender hydrosol	2 ounces (56.7 grams)
Chamomile hydrosol	2 ounces (56.7 grams)

Aloe vera juice	2 ounces (56.7 grams)
Palmarosa essential oil	.08 ounce (2.3 grams)
Vitamin E	1 gel cap
Preservative	(see manufacturer's recommendation)

Prepare as directed in the Facial Toner for Normal to Dry Skin recipe.

The Least You Need to Know

- Always weigh all your ingredients so your recipes will come out correctly.
- Don't forget or skip sterilizing your container and workspace.
- With these recipes, you can make all your own skin care needs—chemical-free!—and save money and be environmentally friendly, too!

Body Beautiful

In This Chapter

- Luscious, pampering body butters
- Wonderful lotions that are a snap to make!
- DIY skin-improving scrubs
- Milk baths, bath bombs, and bath teas to soothe and relax

In this chapter, we take a look at how different oils and butters combine to make wonderful creams, lotions, body butters, bath fizzies, and many more lovely bath and body products.

You might notice that the recipes add up to 102 percent. That's not a typo! We don't include the amount of preservative or scent as part of the 100 percent in these recipes. Scent is optional, and the amount of preservative depends on the type and brand of preservative you're using. I prefer Optiphen Plus for these recipes. It's paraben- and formaldehyde-free, and its use rate is 1 percent. (See Appendix E for more on preservatives.)

Before we begin, let me again stress the importance of cleanliness. *Always* clean your work area with white vinegar or 3 percent hydrogen peroxide before you start working. And be sure to sanitize your containers with alcohol or a commercial sanitizer.

Making Body Butter

Body butters nourish our oil-starved skin in a delicious way. A good body butter will completely soak into your skin within a few minutes after applying it. It shouldn't just sit on top of your skin, leaving you feeling greasy or like a well-buttered turkey ready to go into the oven!

Your skin also should not feel tight or dry an hour after applying the butter. Body butter should leave your skin soft and moisturized all day. Many commercially made body butters and lotions use chemicals such as sodium hydroxide (lye) as thickeners. These can dry out your skin so much that an hour later, you need to reapply.

There are several ways to make body butter. One is to soften the butters and add oil while whipping the mixture with an electric mixer. The problem with this method is that it doesn't hold up very well over time, in shipping, or in a warm climate. We've found that it's much better to make body butter using *emulsifying wax* and stearic acid. This gives you a nice, rich butter that holds together to the very last drop.

BEAUTY BIT

Emulsifying wax (or ewax) is a wax made from vegetable waxes and is used to bind oils and water together to make lotions, creams, and body butters. It's easy to work with.

In these recipes, we've used common but very good butters and oils. By no means are you limited to only these oils and butters—you can swap one butter for a different butter or oil you want to use. As long as you keep the total combined weight of oils and butters the same, the recipe will still work.

Here's what you need to make body butters:

- Stove
- Scale
- Stainless-steel stockpot (6 or 8 quarts)
- Immersion blender
- Long-handled plastic or stainless-steel spoon
- Meat or candy thermometer
- Cereal bowl–size glass or plastic bowl
- Small plastic pitcher
- 2 small glass measuring cups or other type of glass cup
- 4-ounce (113.4-gram), 8-ounce (226.8-gram), or 16-ounce (453.6-gram) jars and bottles

Thick and Luscious Body Butter

This is an incredibly thick and luscious body butter—as the name implies! The butter sinks into your skin quickly within a couple minutes and leaves it feeling soft and moist all day, without feeling sticky or greasy. This recipe makes 32 ounces (907.2 grams), or 8 (4-ounce; 113.4-gram) jars or 4 (8-ounce; 226.8-gram) jars.

Grapeseed oil	2 ounces (56.7 grams)
Sweet almond oil	2.5 ounces (70.9 grams)
Avocado oil	2 ounces (56.7 grams)
Shea butter	2.5 ounces (70.9 grams)
Mango butter	2.5 ounces (70.9 grams)
Cocoa butter	2.25 ounces (63.8 grams)
Kokum (or other butter of choice)	2.25 ounces (63.8 grams)
Emulsifying wax	2 ounces (56.7 grams)
Stearic acid	1 ounce (28.4 grams)
Distilled water	13 ounces (368.5 grams)
Preservative	(see manufacturer's recommendation)
Skin-safe fragrance or essential oil	.3 ounce (8.5 grams)

1. Place the plastic pitcher on the scale, and push the tare button to zero out the weight of the pitcher. Weigh each oil in the pitcher separately and pour into the stainless-steel pot. Place the plastic bowl on the scale, press tare, and repeat the process for each butter.

2. Place the pot over low heat. Let the oils and butters completely melt, stirring occasionally to help the butters melt.

3. Using your thermometer to check the temperature of the combined oils and butters, bring the mixture to 180°F. If you're using unrefined butter, hold the mixture at that temperature for 20 minutes. This kills any germs or bacteria that may be in the unrefined butter. Be careful not to overheat—overheated butter, such as mango and cocoa butter, will crystallize later on and feel grainy.

4. On your scale, weigh out the emulsifying wax and stearic acid and add to the pot. While the wax is melting, weigh out distilled water. Place water in the microwave for 60 seconds at a time until the water is at least 140°F. (The water must be warm before you add it to the mixture.) Add the water to the mixture, and use an immersion blender to bring the oils, wax, and water together to form a good emulsion. Remove from heat and allow to cool to 110°F.

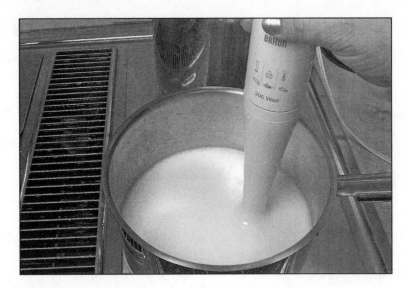

5. Put your glass measuring cup on the scale, push the tare button, and weigh the fragrance oil. Now get another glass cup, put it on the scale, and again push the tare button.

6. When mixture has cooled to 110°F, weigh out and add your preservative and fragrance. Again, use your immersion blender to incorporate all the ingredients. At this time you can also add a skin-safe colorant. Follow the amount recommended by the manufacturer.

7. Let cool completely, and pour into sterile jars.

As the body butter cools, it will thicken into a beautiful, rich, thick butter.

IN THE MIRROR

The women of West and Central Africa depend on the manufacturing and exporting of shea butter. By working with the shea butter, these women have become independent and are able to support and educate their children.

Simple Body Butter

This body butter is simple but very effective. This recipe makes 24 ounces (680.4 grams), or 6 (4-ounce; 113.4-gram) jars or 3 (8-ounce; 226.8-gram) jars.

Sweet almond oil	2 ounces (56.7 grams)
Grapeseed oil	2.8 ounces (79.4 grams)
Shea butter	4 ounces (113.4 grams)
Cocoa butter	2.6 ounces (73.7 grams)
Emulsifying wax	1.9 ounces (53.9 grams)
Stearic acid	.7 ounce (19.8 grams)
Distilled water	10 ounces (283.5 grams)
Preservative	(see manufacturer's recommendation)
Skin-safe fragrance or essential oil	.25 ounce (7.1 grams)

Prepare as directed in the Thick and Luscious Body Butter recipe. Let cool completely, and pour into sterile jars.

Body Butter for Mature Skin

The meadowfoam seed oil in this recipe carries the butters and oils deep through all the layers of the skin, making this a perfect butter for more mature skin. This recipe makes 64 ounces (1,814.4 grams), or 8 (8-ounce; 226.8-gram) jars or 16 (4-ounce; 113.4-gram) jars.

Sweet almond oil	8.5 ounces (241 grams)
Evening primrose oil	4 ounces (113.4 grams)
Pumpkin seed oil	2 ounces (56.7 grams)
Meadowfoam seed oil	4.5 ounces (127.6 grams)
Unrefined shea butter	8.5 ounces (241 grams)
Cocoa butter	5.5 ounces (155.9 grams)
Emulsifying wax	5 ounces (141.7 grams)
Stearic acid	2 ounces (56.7 grams)
Distilled water	24 ounces (680.4 grams)
Preservative	(see manufacturer's recommendation)
Skin-safe fragrance or essential oil	.6 ounce (17 grams)

Prepare as directed in the Thick and Luscious Body Butter recipe. Let cool completely, and pour into sterile jars.

Pregnant Belly Butter

I created this recipe for my daughter while she was pregnant. During her pregnancies, she applied the butter several times a day and happily has only a few small stretch marks after having had three babies. Since then, whenever one of her friends becomes pregnant, they come to me for this butter. Remember, many essential oils can be harmful to children and pregnant women, so please don't use essential oils in this butter. This recipe makes 32 ounces (907.2 grams), or 4 (8-ounce; 226.8-gram) jars or 8 (4-ounce; 113.4-gram) jars.

Sweet almond oil	3 ounces (85 grams)
Peach kernel oil	3.5 ounces (99.2 grams)
Meadowfoam seed oil	2.5 ounces (70.9 grams)
Cocoa butter	4 ounces (113.4 grams)
Shea butter	3 ounces (85 grams)
Emulsifying wax	2.5 ounces (70.9 grams)
Stearic acid	1 ounce (28.4 grams)
Distilled water	12.5 ounces (354.4 grams)
Preservative	(see manufacturer's recommendation)
Skin-safe fragrance oil	.3 ounce (8.5 grams)

Prepare as directed in the Thick and Luscious Body Butter recipe. Let cool completely, and pour into jars.

Only-the-Best Body Butter

Only the best oils and butters are used in this rich and decadent butter, and your skin will welcome it and drink it in. A few of the oils and butters in this recipe are a little pricey, but they are so worth it! Do practice by making the other recipes before you tackle this one. It's not hard, but we wouldn't want you to start out making butters for the first time using these more expensive oils and butters. This recipe makes 32 ounces (907.2 grams), or 4 (8-ounce; 226.8-gram) jars or 8 (4-ounce; 113.4-gram) jars.

Kukui oil	2.5 ounces (70.9 grams)
Peach kernel oil	2.5 ounces (70.9 grams)
Evening primrose oil	1.5 ounces (42.5 grams)
Illipe butter	2 ounces (56.7 grams)
Cupuacu butter	5 ounces (141.7 grams)
Cocoa butter	2 ounces (56.7 grams)

Emulsifying wax	2.5 ounces (70.9 grams)
Stearic acid	1 ounce (28.4 grams)
Distilled water	12.5 ounces (354.4 grams)
Preservative	(see manufacturer's recommendation)
Skin-safe fragrance or essential oil	.3 ounce (8.5 grams)

Prepare as directed in the Thick and Luscious Body Butter recipe. Let cool completely, and pour into sterile jars.

> **IN THE MIRROR**
>
> The fruit of the Cupuacu tree provides a wonderful butter. Cupuacu butter hydrates very dry skin and hair, returning its natural softness and smoothness. This butter can be used in place of lanolin in products and is a good vegetable alternative. This body butter is wonderful for cancer patients who are going through chemotherapy, especially since chemo is so drying. Cancer patients are often nauseated by smells, so avoid using any scent in a body butter or lotion for them.

Painful Feet Cream

The arnica herb, which helps ease pain, is often infused in oil and used in lotions, balms, and sticks. Rub your feet with this cream after a long day, and in no time you'll realize your feet are no longer aching. You won't feel heat or cold like you do from commercial muscle rubs and such. This recipe makes 32 ounces (907.2 grams), or 4 (8-ounce; 226.8-gram) jars or 8 (4-ounce; 113.4-gram) jars.

Meadowfoam seed oil	2.5 ounces (70.9 grams)
Sunflower oil double infused with arnica (herb)	6.5 ounces (184.3 grams)
Shea butter	3.5 ounces (99.2 grams)
Cocoa butter	3.5 ounces (99.2 grams)
Emulsifying wax	2.5 ounces (70.9 grams)
Stearic acid	1 ounce (28.4 grams)
Distilled water	12.5 ounces (354.4 grams)
Preservative	(see manufacturer's recommendation)
Peppermint essential oil	.3 ounce (8.5 grams)

Prepare as directed in the Thick and Luscious Body Butter recipe. Let cool completely, and pour into jars.

Antifungal Cream

This cream really works! If you have smelly feet, all you have to do is rub this cream on your feet every morning, and your feet will stay fresh and odor-free all day long. You can also use this under your arms instead of using a commercial deodorant. This recipe makes 24 ounces (680.4 grams), or 4 (8-ounce; 226.8-gram) jars or 8 (4-ounce; 113.4-gram) jars.

Black cumin seed oil	3.6 ounces (102.1 grams)
Karanja oil	2.9 ounces (82.2 grams)
Neem oil	1.5 ounces (42.5 grams)
Emu oil	2.9 ounces (82.2 grams)
Emulsifying wax	1.9 ounces (53.9 grams)
Stearic acid	.8 ounce (22.7 grams)
Aloe vera gel (used in place of water)	9.4 ounces (266.5 grams)
Preservative	(see manufacturer's recommendation)
Essential oil blend	1 ounce (28.4 grams)

For the essential oil blend, use equal parts (.14 ounce; 4 grams) of these essential oils:

German chamomile	Eucalyptus
Lemongrass	Peppermint
Rosemary	Thyme
Cinnamon or clove	

Prepare as directed in the Thick and Luscious Body Butter recipe. Let cool completely, and pour into sterile jars.

SAFETY FIRST

Many people find cinnamon essential oil causes skin irritation. If you use it, use a lesser percentage. And I love the smell of peppermint, but it also can cause a burning sensation on the skin. Use both of these essential oils with care.

Making Lotions

You make lotions the same way you make body butters. However, they are very different from body butters. Lotions have a thinner and lighter consistency. The oil and butter ratio is less in lotions than it is in body butters. And in lotion, the water ratio is higher, which is why the body butters are so much richer and thicker than lotions.

Lotions are for light moisturizing, and body butters are for deep moisturizing. Just follow the body butter directions given earlier, and you'll have perfect lotion every time.

If, after your lotion has completely cooled, it's too thin, you can fix that. Simply reheat it to 110°F and add another 1 percent of the mixture's total weight of the melted emulsifying wax. Use the immersion blender to incorporate the emulsifying wax, and let it totally cool again. Repeat until the lotion is as thick as you want.

PRETTY POINTER

Really love one of the lotion recipes, or not sure you'll like it enough to use a whole batch? You're in luck! Each of the lotion recipes can be cut in half to make a smaller batch or doubled if you want more.

Baby Lotion

This lotion is very gentle and soothing, and the cocoa butter helps protect baby's young, tender skin. Remember, using essential oils on babies is not recommended, so choose a fragrance oil instead. This recipe makes 32 ounces (907.2 grams), or 4 (8-ounce; 226.8-gram) jars or 8 (4-ounce; 113.4-gram) bottles.

Sunflower oil single infused with calendula (herb)	2 ounces (56.7 grams)
Sunflower oil single infused with chamomile (herb)	2 ounces (56.7 grams)
Cocoa butter	.4 ounce (11.3 grams)
Emulsifying wax	1.6 ounces (45.4 grams)
Distilled water	24 ounces (680.4 grams)
Aloe vera gel	2 ounces (56.7 grams)
Preservative	(see manufacturer's recommendation)
Skin-safe fragrance oil	.3 ounce (8.5 grams)

Prepare as directed in the Thick and Luscious Body Butter recipe. Let cool completely, and pour into sterile jars.

PRETTY POINTER

Oregon Trails has a soft baby fragrance called Sweet Innocence that I often use for this recipe.

Light and Silky Lotion

I love this lotion for quick applications during the day when I've been washing my hands a lot. It's just enough to replace the moisture in my hands without making them slippery. You can cut this recipe in half to make a smaller batch, or you can double it—or even double it several times—to make larger batches. This recipe makes 64 ounces (1,814.4 grams), or 4 (16-ounce; 453.6-gram) jars or 8 (8-ounce; 226.8-gram) bottles.

Sweet almond oil	6.5 ounces (184.3 grams)
Peach kernel oil	3 ounces (85 grams)
Avocado oil	2.5 ounce (70.9 grams)
Cocoa butter	.8 ounce (22.7 grams)
Emulsifying wax	3.2 ounces (90.7 grams)
Distilled water	48 ounces (1,360.8 grams)
Preservative	(see manufacturer's recommendation)
Skin-safe fragrance oil	.6 ounce (17 grams)

Prepare as directed in the Thick and Luscious Body Butter recipe. Let cool completely, and pour into sterile bottles.

Light and Lovely Lotion

This lotion is light yet gives you enough moisturizing to last all day. Make a gallon and give as holiday gifts to your family and friends or dole out as party favors. You can also halve this recipe as many times as you want to make a smaller batch. This recipe makes 128 ounces (3,628.7 grams), or 8 (16-ounce; 453.6-gram) bottles or 16 (8-ounce; 226.8-gram) bottles or 32 (4-ounce; 113.4-gram) bottles.

Sweet almond oil	6 ounces (170.1 grams)
Grapeseed oil	8 ounces (226.8 grams)
Apricot kernel oil	6 ounces (170.1 grams)
Peach kernel oil	5.5 ounces (155.9 grams)
Cocoa butter	6 ounces (170.1 grams)
Emulsifying wax	6.5 ounces (184.3 grams)
Distilled water	90 ounces (2,551.5 grams)
Preservative	(see manufacturer's recommendation)
Skin-safe fragrance or essential oil	1.3 ounces (36.9 grams)

Prepare as directed in the Thick and Luscious Body Butter recipe. Let cool completely, and pour into sterile bottles.

Super-Rich Lotion for Mature Skin

This is my favorite recipe! I use this lotion every day. Use it once a day, and your skin will stay soft and moist all day long. This recipe makes 16 ounces (453.6 grams), or 1 (16-ounce; 453.6-gram) bottle or 2 (8-ounce; 226.8-gram) bottles.

Pumpkin seed oil	.5 ounce (14.2 grams)
Peach kernel oil	2 ounces (56.7 grams)
Evening primrose oil	2 ounces (56.7 grams)
Flaxseed oil	.5 ounce (14.2 grams)
Shea butter (cosmetic grade)	2 ounces (56.7 grams)
Emulsifying wax	1 ounce (28.4 grams)
Distilled water	8 ounces (226.8 grams)
Preservative	(see manufacturer's recommendation)
Skin-safe fragrance or essential oil	.15 ounce (4.3 grams)

Prepare as directed in the Thick and Luscious Body Butter recipe. Let cool completely, and pour into sterile bottles.

Moisturizer for Acne-Prone Skin

Just because you have acne or problem skin doesn't mean your skin never needs moisturizing. Jojoba oil is very similar to our own natural sebum, so it "tricks" our body into producing so much sebum, which helps clear the skin. Plus, jojoba oil doesn't aggravate acne. This lotion gives just enough moisture to the skin to keep it soft. It's also an excellent makeup remover! This recipe makes 4 ounces (113.4 grams), or 2 (2-ounce; 56.7-gram) bottles.

Jojoba oil	4 ounces (113.4 grams)
Lavender essential oil	.04 ounce (1.2 milliliters; 30 drops)
Tea tree essential oil	.02 ounce (.6 milliliter; 10 drops)

1. Weigh the oil and add the essential oils.

2. Shake well and pour into a sterile bottle or bottles. Shake well again before each use.

Making Body Powders

Body powders are nice and soothing, especially during the warm months. You can use several types of natural powders as a base. Cornstarch and baking soda are inexpensive and readily available in your local drugstore or grocery store.

Body powders are so easy to make, and because they're very lightweight, 4 ounces (113.4 grams)—which is what these recipes make—is a lot of powder!

You don't need a lot of tools to make body powders:

- Large mixing bowl
- Scale
- Latex gloves
- Shaker containers or jars

SAFETY FIRST

Please wear latex gloves while mixing with your hands. Even if you wash your hands very thoroughly, there might still be germs and bacteria on your skin.

Simple After-Bath Powder

Using an after-bath powder helps keep you feeling fresh and dry for hours after you've showered. This is a basic recipe you can add your own touches and tweaks to. This recipe makes 24 ounces (680.4 grams), or 3 (8-ounce; 226.8-gram) jars or shakers or 6 (4-ounce; 113.4-gram) jars or shakers.

Cornstarch	4 ounces (113.4 grams)
Arrowroot	4 ounces (113.4 grams)
Baking soda	8 ounces (226.8 grams)
Tapioca starch	8 ounces (226.8 grams)
Fragrance oil or essential oil	1 teaspoon (4.9 milliliters)

1. Put a bowl on the scale and push the tare button to zero out the weight of the bowl. Weigh each of your ingredients, and place them in a large bowl.

2. Use your hands to thoroughly mix all the dry ingredients.

3. Place a small glass or stainless-steel cup on the scale, and push the tare button to zero out the weight of the cup. Weigh your fragrance oil.

4. Drizzle the fragrance slowly into the dry mixture, again using your hands to work it into the powder mixture.

5. Package the powder in a sterile shaker container or a sterile jar that has a lid.

PRETTY POINTER

For the essential oil blend, try using lemon, sweet orange, and lime essential oils. Yum!

Making Scrubs

Scrubs are excellent for exfoliating your whole body. You can use them in the bathtub or shower to remove dead skin cells and make your whole body feel silky soft.

There are several ways to make scrubs. You can keep the sugar and oils separate and only mix them when you're ready to use them, you can mix everything together at once, or you can emulsify the sugar and oils. Whichever technique you choose to use, I'm sure you'll agree that sugar scrubs leave your skin feeling soft and silky to the touch.

In all these recipes, you can use sea salt in place of sugar. Please don't use salt in a scrub meant to be used on the face, however. Salt can be too abrasive for the facial skin, and it might lead to you scheduling an appointment with your dermatologist.

Here's what you need to make scrubs:

- Large mixing bowl
- Small stainless-steel stockpot
- Spoons
- Electric mixer
- Scale
- Several plastic containers for storage
- Small glass or stainless-steel cup
- Stove or microwave

Wow! What a Scrub

This is my favorite sugar scrub. You'll love the way it leaves your skin feeling. I formulated this scrub several years ago when I first started teaching classes and used this recipe in those first lessons. This recipe makes 32 ounces (907.2 grams), or 4 (8-ounce; 226.8-gram) jars or 8 (4-ounce; 113.4-gram) jars.

Sweet almond oil	2 ounces (56.7 grams)
Grapeseed oil	2 ounces (56.7 grams)
Jojoba oil	1 ounce (28.4 grams)
Apricot kernel oil	2 ounces (56.7 grams)
Emulsifying wax	3.3 ounces (93.6 grams)
Stearic acid	2.2 ounces (62.4 grams)
Cocoa butter	2.5 ounces (70.9 grams)
Shea butter	1 ounce (28.4 grams)
White or brown sugar	16 ounces (453.6 grams)
Preservative	(see manufacturer's recommendation)
Skin-safe fragrance or essential oil	.3 ounce (8.5 grams)

1. Put a bowl on the scale and push the tare button to zero out the weight of the bowl. Weigh each of your oils, and place them in a bowl to be added later.

2. Place the bowl back on the scale and push the tare button again. Weigh the emulsifying wax, stearic acid, cocoa butter, and shea butter.

3. Place the waxes and butters in a small stockpot and place over low heat.

4. When the wax and butter have melted, add the oils. You can hand-stir this or use your immersion blender to bring the oils and wax together. Let cool for about 30 minutes.

5. Return to the scale and place the bowl back on the top. Push the tare button to zero out the weight of the bowl. Now weigh your sugar.

6. Add the sugar to the pot of cooled oils and stir well. Let completely cool. Using an electric mixer, whip the scrub for about 5 minutes until it is thick and fluffy.

7. Package in sterile jars or other airtight sterile containers.

Simple Sugar Scrub

Have you ever treated yourself to a sugar scrub in the tub or shower? You should! It's amazing how soft and silky your skin feels afterward. The sugar gently removes dead skin, and the oils soften and rejuvenate the new skin under all the dead cells. This basic recipe gets you started—and most likely hooked on sugar scrubs for life! This recipe makes 26 ounces (737.1 grams).

Oil (your choice)	6 ounces (170.1 grams)
White or brown sugar	16 ounces (453.6 grams)
Finely ground oatmeal	4 ounces (113.4 grams)
Preservative	(see manufacturer's recommendation)
Fragrance oil	.3 ounce (8.5 grams)

Prepare as directed in the Wow! What a Scrub recipe.

Making Shower Scrub Cubes

Recently these fun little scrub cubes have become very popular among home-crafters. These one-time-use shower scrub cubes fit into the palm of your hand, making them easy to use in the shower. Wet your skin and then rub the sugar scrub cube all over your body. Wait a few minutes before you completely rinse. It's as simple as that!

(Note: I didn't create this recipe; it was given to me by another soap-maker.)

Here's what you need to make shower scrub cubes:

- Small stainless-steel saucepan or microwaveable container
- Scale
- 1 large bowl and 1 smaller bowl
- Several spoons
- Stove or microwave
- Electric mixer
- A 6×6-inch plastic square container or a small muffin tin (You might want to try using a meatball maker, but you'd have to work quickly before the scrub sets up.)
- Zipper-lock bags, 6×6 foil candy wrappers, or cello bags

Shower Scrub Cubes

These are fun to make and wonderful to use! Because we use melt-and-pour soap, this recipe makes a great and fun project to use with children. We did not formulate this recipe, just tweaked it a little. For fun, try adding a few drops of skin-safe colorant. This recipe makes 24 (1-ounce; 28.4-gram) shower scrub cubes or 12 (2-ounce; 56.7-gram) cubes.

Oil(s) (your choice)	5 ounces (141.7 grams)
Clear melt-and-pour glycerin soap base	5 ounces (141.7 grams)
White or brown sugar	14 ounces (396.9 grams)
Fragrance or essential oil	.6 ounce (17 grams)
Preservative	(see manufacturer's recommendation)

1. Place a bowl on the scale and push the tare button. Weigh the first oil. Place it in another bowl. Put the bowl back on the scale and push the tare button again and weigh the next oil. Continue until you've weighed all your oils.

2. Place the bowl on the scales again and push tare. Weigh the melt-and-pour soap. Place the soap in a small saucepan, and set over low heat. Be careful not to get the soap too hot.

3. Once again place the bowl on the scale, and push the tare button. Weigh the sugar. Set it aside for now.

4. Once the soap base is completely melted, add the oils, sugar, and fragrance oil. Use an electric mixer to whip it all together.

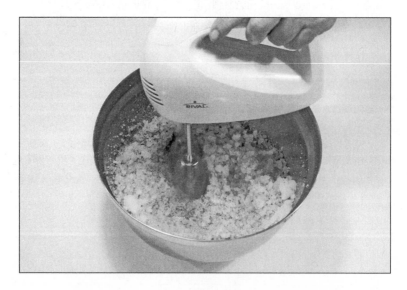

5. Add the preservative and colorant (if desired).

6. Spoon into the plastic container, smooth out flat, and press firmly, or spoon into the muffin pan and press firmly.

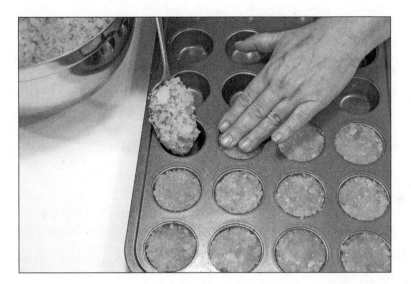

7. Let set up for a few minutes and then, if in square container, cut into even-size squares. Set out on waxed paper to continue hardening. If you used a muffin tin, gently remove the cubes from tin and continue to let harden on waxed paper.

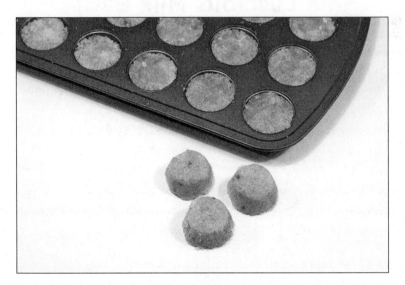

> **PRETTY POINTER**
>
> To add a little more oomph to this scrub, instead of a single oil, try blending sweet almond oil, grapeseed oil, and apricot kernel oil. You can use equal parts or more or less of the oils. And if you use white sugar, you can also use a few drops of food coloring or skin-safe colorant to color the cubes.

Making Milk Baths

Milk baths are very simple to make. And I use the powdered milk from the grocery store to make it even easier! All you have to do is weigh the ingredients, pour them into your bowl, mix it all together, and you're done! Store the bath in a plastic container or in cello bags. Add ½ cup (115 grams) of milk bath to your bathwater.

Here's what you need to make milk baths:

- Large mixing bowl
- Spoon
- Scale
- Latex gloves
- Large food-type airtight plastic container or cello bags

Luscious Milk Bath

We have always heard about the benefits of milk baths. This is a simple and quick recipe for making a powdered milk bath you will surely love. Package in cello bags and give as gifts to your friends and family. Or use an airtight container and keep by your bathtub for those special "me" times. This recipe makes 42.5 ounces (1,204.9 grams).

Powdered milk	16 ounces (453.6 grams)
Baking soda	16 ounces (453.6 grams)
Cornstarch	8 ounces (226.8 grams)
Sweet almond oil (or your choice)	2 ounces (56.7 grams)
Preservative	(see manufacturer's recommendation)
Skin-safe fragrance oil	.4 ounce (11.3 grams)

1. Place a bowl on the scale and push the tare button. Weigh all the dry ingredients one at a time and put them in a mixing bowl. Set aside. Remember to push the tare button each time you place the bowl back on the scale.

2. Weigh the liquids the same way you did the dry ingredients. Drizzle the liquids into the dry mixture.

3. Using your hands (and wearing latex gloves), mix everything together until the liquids are well distributed throughout the mixture.

4. Package in cello bags or in an airtight container.

Making Bath Tea

Bath teas are made by blending several dried herbs and packaging them in heat-sealable tea bags or in muslin drawstring bags. If you use muslin bags, you'll need to refill them before each use. To use, simply toss a tea bag in the tub while the bath-water is running. If you're using the muslin bags, you can hang them over the water faucet under the running water as the tub fills. Then just leave the tea bag in the tub while you soak and bathe.

Here's what you need to make bath teas:

- Scale
- 1 large bowl and 1 small bowl
- Latex gloves
- Large sealable tea bags or muslin bags
- Spoon
- Iron

Floral Bath Tea

Relax in a warm tub of water while enjoying the blended fragrance of roses, lavender, chamomile, and calendula. Let the fragrance carry you back to warm summer days in the garden. This recipe makes 16 ounces (453.6 grams).

Dried rose buds	4 ounces (113.4 grams)
Dried lavender buds	4 ounces (113.4 grams)
Dried chamomile flowers	4 ounces (113.4 grams)
Dried calendula flowers	4 ounces (113.4 grams)

1. Place a bowl on your scale and push the tare button. Weigh your dried flowers one at a time, and place them in a large bowl. Remember to push the tare button after you replace your bowl each time.

2. Wearing latex gloves on your hands, mix all the flowers together.

3. If you're using the large sealable tea bags, scoop out about 1 tablespoon (14.8 milliliters) and place it in the middle of one side of the flat bag. Fold the bag over and line up the edges. Use an iron on low setting to seal the edges of the tea bags.

If using muslin bags, scoop out about ¼ cup (59.2 milliliters) and fill the muslin bag. Draw the string tight, and tie in a tiny knot.

> **PRETTY POINTER**
>
> You can make a large batch of tea bags and store them in an airtight container until you're ready to use them.

Making Bath Oils

I love making bath oils, and I love using them even more! For my bath oils, I always use Turkey red oil (red castor oil) because it won't leave a ring around the tub. If you have an herb garden, you're going to have lots of fun infusing your herbs in the oils to make incredible herbal bath oils. These make wonderful gifts, too! When ready to use, just pour about ½ ounce (14.2 grams) of oil in your tub as you fill it with water.

Here's what you need to make bath oils:

- Scale
- Sterile bottles
- Funnel
- Small glass or stainless-steel cup

Lavender Bath Oil

This bath oil is very good for children who have attention deficit/hyperactivity disorder (ADHD). It relaxes them and helps them get a better night's sleep, which means a better day tomorrow. My grandson Shawn had a warm lavender bath every night. It calmed him and he would be ready for bed the minute he got out of the tub. Use 1 ounce (28.4 grams) to ½ ounce (14.2 grams) per warm bath. This recipe makes just over 8 ounces (226.8 grams).

Turkey red oil	6 ounces (170.1 grams)
Sweet almond oil (or your choice)	2 ounces (56.7 grams)

| Lavender essential oil | .2 ounce (5.7 grams) |
| Preservative | (see manufacturer's recommendation) |

1. Place a small measuring cup on the scale and push the tare button to zero out the weight of the cup. Weigh the Turkey red oil.

2. Using the funnel, pour the oil into a sterile 8-ounce (226.8-gram) bottle. Scrape as much of the oil as you can out of the cup.

3. Put the cup back on the scale and once again push the tare button. Weigh the next oil and again use the funnel to pour it into the bottle. Repeat until all the oils have been poured into the bottle, including the scent and preservative.

4. Shake the bottle to mix all the oils together completely. Put the lid on it, and you are done!

Basic Bath Oil

In this basic bath oil recipe, you can choose your own scent or scent blend. (We've listed a few blends for you to try in the next section.) You can also blend your favorite oils to make this recipe more your own. Just keep the ratios the same. You can double this as many times as you like to make the batch size you want. This recipe makes 8 ounces (226.8 grams).

Turkey red oil	6 ounces (170.1 grams)
Sweet almond oil	1 ounce (28.4 grams)
Grapeseed oil	1 ounce (28.4 grams)
Skin-safe fragrance oil	.2 ounce (5.7 grams)
Preservative	(see manufacturer's recommendation)

Prepare as directed in the Lavender Bath Oil recipe.

Making Fragrance Blends

On our Yahoo! group, ApplesNBerries, we are lucky to have Alex Crow, a.k.a. "the happy blender," who is well known for his blending skills. Alex has written many articles for "Cowboy's Corner," part of the Apples, Woods and Berries website. He has graciously given us permission to include a few of his wonderful blends so you can enjoy using them to make your bath oil very special. Alex has also written an e-book explaining how to make your own fragrance oil blends.

These recipes are all written in "parts" so you can make the blend in the amount you need for your project. One part can be anything from 1 teaspoon (4.9 milliliters) to 1 pound (453.6 grams) or even more.

These blends, all made using fragrance oils, are suitable for all bath and body products and soap.

Moonlit Tango Fragrance Blend

Soft floral, but with sweet notes from the hibiscus, this blend is very light and airy.

1 part moonlight path   1 part hibiscus

St. Louis Slide Fragrance Blend

Creamy caramel and vanilla from Crème Brûlée pair well with the tart notes of pomegranate.

2 parts crème brûlée   1 part pomegranate

English Porcelain Fragrance Blend

English heather is grounded by the bottom notes of soft and spicy myrrh.

2 parts myrrh   1 part English heather

Christmas Rose Fragrance Blend

This blend captures the magic of a spicy white rose, blooming in the frost.

2 parts white roses   1 part holiday memories

Pearl of the East Fragrance Blend

The soft floral of the cherry blossom and the sensuous warmth of sandalwood make this an exotic blend.

2 parts sandalwood   1 part white cherry blossom

Making Bath Bombs

Bath bombs are a fun way to add a few skin-softening ingredients and fragrance to your bath. When tossed in a tub of water, they fizz until they've dissolved. Children love them, but they're not only for children—us big kids love them, too!

Making bath bombs can be very frustrating at times. I've made beautiful bombs, laid them out to dry, and then had them start growing because it rained or it became too humid. I have smooshed them into candy molds and used a meat baller to form perfect balls, but my best success has been with the bath bomb tapper. You can find them online for around $6.

All bath bombs are made pretty much the same. There's very little difference among recipes. Play with the recipe we've given you, and find the oil and molding method you prefer. You may or may not want to dry them in your oven. It's purely a matter of what process you like best.

Here's what you'll need to make bath bombs:

- Large stainless-steel bowl
- Electric mixer
- Small jar with lid
- Cookie sheet
- Latex gloves
- Mold, either a candy mold or a bath bomb tapper
- 6×6 foil candy wrappers
- Colorant (optional)

Bath Bomb

This is a basic recipe for bath bombs used by many hand-crafters. We learned a trick from Sandra Morrow that's made a huge difference in how well our bombs turn out: she taught us to hold the citric acid back from the mixture until the liquid has already been well mixed in. This stops the fizzing that would happen when the liquid was added. 100 percent improvement! This recipe makes 24 ounces (680.4 grams), or 12 (2-ounce; 56.7-gram) bombs or 24 (1-ounce; 28.4-gram) bombs.

Citric acid   8 ounces (226.8 grams)
(Save the citric acid to add
after you've added the liquid.)

The dry ingredients:

Cornstarch	8 ounces (226.8 grams)
Baking soda	16 ounces (453.6 grams)

The wet ingredients:

Sweet almond oil	.5 ounce (14.2 grams)
Turkey red oil (red castor oil)	.5 ounce (14.2 grams)
Distilled water	½ teaspoon (2.5 milliliters)
Fragrance or essential oil	1 teaspoon (4.9 milliliters)
Skin-safe colorant, if desired	½ teaspoon (2.5 milliliters)

1. Place a bowl on your scale and push the tare button. Weigh the citric acid, and set it aside for now.

2. Weigh the cornstarch and place it in the large bowl. Repeat this with the baking soda. Mix together and set aside.

3. Measure the wet ingredients and pour into the small jar. If you're adding colorant, add it to this mixture in the small jar. Screw the lid on the jar, and shake it.

4. Slowly drizzle the wet ingredients into the dry ingredients, and stir for a minute. With an electric mixer on low, mix for several minutes to ensure the wet ingredients are evenly incorporated into the dry ingredients.

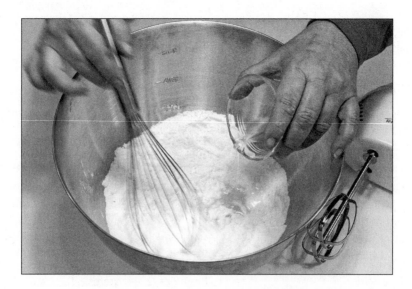

5. Add the citric acid, and continue mixing to distribute the citric acid throughout the bath bomb mixture.

6. Press the bomb mixture into a candy mold or use the bath bomb tapper to form your bath bombs. They don't need to sit very long in a candy mold, but if they're not packed tight enough, they sometimes fall apart when turned out on a cookie sheet. Arrange your bombs on a cookie sheet.

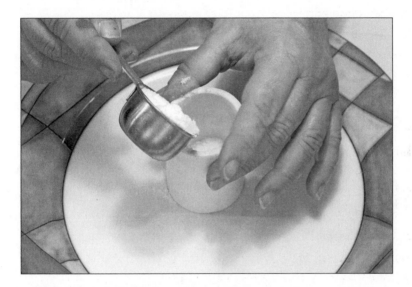

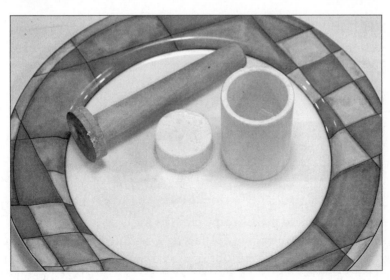

7. Preheat the oven to 170°F or the lowest setting. When the oven is hot, *turn it off,* and place the cookie sheet with bombs in the oven. Close the door and let sit for 1 hour to harden and dry the bombs.

8. Remove bombs from the oven and let sit for several days to dry completely. Wrap each bath bomb in a candy foil.

IN THE MIRROR

Why are the ingredients for this recipe measured in teaspoons and milliliters rather than ounces? Quite simply, because they're old recipes and no one has ever changed from this method. When it works, we leave it as it is!

Making Jelly Soap for Kids

My grandchildren love this slippery, floppy jelly soap. It's easy to make and fun for them to use. Simply store it in an airtight container in the refrigerator and break off a piece for the kids at bath time. (Note: I did not create this recipe; it was given to me by another soap-maker.)

Here's what you need to make jelly soap:

- Bowl
- Scale
- Saucepan or microwavable container
- Teakettle or microwavable container
- Stove or microwave
- Spoon
- Square plastic container for mold

Bath-Time Jelly Soap for Kids

This is another recipe that's fun for children to make and even more fun for them to use. Use cookie cutters to make creepy crawlies for little boys, and watch them happily run to the tub with their "bug." Add a dash of fine glitter and colorant to make it pretty for the little girls in your life. This bath jelly soap makes bath time loads of fun—and big kids like it, too! This recipe makes 22 ounces (623.7 grams).

Unflavored gelatin	1 (¼-ounce; 7.1-gram) envelope
Boiling water	16 ounces (453.6 grams)
Clear melt-and-pour soap base or clear liquid soap	4 ounces (113.4 grams)
Fragrance oil	.5 ounce (17.2 grams)
Preservative	(see manufacturer's recommendation)
Several skin-safe colorants or food coloring	few drops

1. Pour the gelatin in the bowl and set aside.

2. Weigh 16 ounces (453.6 grams) water and bring to a boil in a tea kettle over medium heat or in a microwave. Slowly pour water into the bowl with the gelatin. Gently stir mixture as it sets up.

3. Weigh and melt the melt-and-pour soap in a saucepan over low heat or in the microwave oven, using short, 1-minute spurts until the soap base has completely melted. Continue to stir the gelatin and water.

4. Add the melt-and-pour soap to the bowl with the gelatin. Add fragrance and preservative, and stir well.

5. Pour the soap into the mold. Add your colorants, and swirl them around in the soap. Place uncovered container in the refrigerator until firm.

6. Remove container and cut into bar shapes or little pieces. You can even use a cookie cutter to cut shapes. Store in an airtight container in the refrigerator.

The Least You Need to Know

- Bath products can be fun to make and relaxing to use—especially when you make them yourself!
- Don't forget that these products will need preservatives. Use Appendix E to help you choose the right preservative for the bath products you're making.
- After you've made the bath product you want to use first, find a few candles for the bathroom and turn on some soothing music. It will revive you after a busy day!

Creating Mineral Makeup

Part 3 is all about makeup, and you'll find recipes for everything you need to look your best in the following chapters.

We start off with the easy-to-follow color grinds for foundations. Our mineral makeup foundation is so light you won't even notice it on your skin, yet it offers superb coverage. Then we share recipes for making concealers and correctors, followed by lots of bronzers and blushes—three color tones for every color group. Next, we look at eyes. You'll find beautiful color grinds for all sorts of eye shadows, and from there, you learn to make eyeliners and mascara. Finally, we "read your lips": with recipes for lipstick, balms, and more, all with loads of luscious color grinds for every color group.

In all, we give you more than 80 color grinds for lips, eyes, and cheeks in Part 3. Once you have learned how to make color grinds using our recipes, you will be able to create your own colors.

Mineral Makeup

In This Chapter

- Making color grinds for your perfect shade
- DIY foundations
- Covering things up with color correctors and concealers
- Pressing your mineral makeup

Once you try mineral makeup, you'll understand why so many women love it. It's so light, it feels like you have *nothing* on your face, yet it stays on your skin until you take it off. I love the natural look mineral makeup provides. For more mature women like me, the mineral makeup lays *over* our fine lines instead of *in* them. That gives us all a younger appearance. Mineral makeup is also more forgiving than commercial foundations because you don't have to match your skin tone as closely.

This all sounds wonderful, doesn't it? It is, as you'll soon see.

The Basics of Making Mineral Makeup

It took about 2 years to work out the color grinds for the foundation and another year or so to perfect the grinds for the blush, bronzer, eye shadow, and lipstick recipes in this book. (See Chapter 9 for more on blushes and bronzers, Chapter 10 for more on eye shadows, and Chapter 11 for more on lipsticks.) Experimenting certainly can get frustrating—during the early days, everything had an orange color, and the foundations definitely had that Bozo the Clown look. Then it all went to the far side and was too yellow. Finally, it all came together.

This chapter is full of what we've learned from our experiences. We share the basic blend tones, called *color grinds*, so you can match your skin type and create your perfect shade. It won't be hard because you have all the formulas and directions we've worked out to help you. You may have to blend several of the grinds together to achieve the exact shade you want, but that's just part of the fun!

Many of these recipes are in several parts. You make your color grind and then you make your base filler, which is white, separately. When you have both made, you add a percentage of the color grind to a percentage of the base filler, grind them together, and you have your foundation!

BEAUTY BIT

Color grinds are micas and oxides blended together by "grinding" in an electric coffee grinder or with a mortar and pestle to create a new color. The micas and oxides have to be very finely ground together.

Here's what you need to make mineral makeup:

- 30-gram shifter jars
- Scale (one that weighs to the 100th is great)
- Measuring spoons and small scoops
- 3mm pipettes
- Face mask
- Latex gloves
- Waxed paper
- Coffee grinder or mortar and pestle
- 6-inch dowel rods the diameter of your containers (for making pressed powder) or TKB Trading pressing tools

IN THE MIRROR

A Mr. Coffee brand coffee grinder blends the oxides and micas quickly and completely. It's inexpensive—about $20—and easy to clean. Get a second grinder if you want to use one for food. For safety, keep one only for your mineral makeup. And you might be wondering if you can use eyedroppers instead of pipettes. You could, but they're difficult to clean for the next use.

In the time since I started writing this book, Kaila at TKB Trading has stocked some very helpful pressing tools and also a liquid binder for pressing. This can replace the extra drops of jojoba oil. I couldn't wait to get my hands on the pressing tools, so as soon as they came in I ordered several sizes. She has added pressing ribbon, too. It not only makes a professional-looking finish on the top of the product, but also helps cut down on the mess. Of course I had to have that, too! I love them both, and I recommend you try them—soon!

Your Work Area

Before we continue, we must reinforce the importance of keeping your work area clean and sanitizing all your containers. Even if these products are only for yourself, you still need to have everything bacteria-free and also use a preservative that kills bacteria and germs. You don't want to end up with a skin or eye infection because of an unknown bacteria in your makeup!

You can use white vinegar or 3 percent hydrogen peroxide to clean your workspace. Neither will leave any harmful chemicals that could accidentally contaminate your cosmetics.

Before you start making anything, wipe your counter or workspace with a clean rag or paper towel soaked in vinegar or hydrogen peroxide. Then place a piece of waxed paper on your work area to help make cleanup quick and easy.

Wash all your containers, spoons, knives, and any other equipment you'll use with hot, soapy water. Let them air-dry. When they're dry, clean the inside of jars, lids, and other containers with alcohol. Let them air-dry again. When they're dry, put them in a zipper-lock bag until you're ready to use them.

I also keep a roll of paper towels and a bottle of alcohol right next to me while I'm working so I can wipe a spoon or a knife when needed. You can never be too clean when making beauty products!

SAFETY FIRST

When making cosmetics, be sure to wear a dust mask and latex gloves. You can accidently breathe in the dust from the micas, oxides, and fine powders. Also, even though you've washed your hands, they may still have germs on the surface. Better to be safe now than sorry later!

Making Pressed Powders

The very name *pressed powder* indicates you'll need to *press* it somehow. In this case, you press it firmly into the container. You pack it in so it's almost a solid. To do this, you need a tamper, or something to gently pound down the powder. We've found a wooden dowel rod works best for this. This will mean a trip to your local hardware store. Take your empty container with you so you can get the correct size dowel.

Look for a dowel that's the same diameter as your container. It needs to fit snugly into the jar without much wiggle room around the sides. Then find a store employee and ask him or her to cut your dowel into 6-inch pieces. This gives you separate dowels for each powder color so you don't have to mix the dowels and risk ruining the color.

SAFETY FIRST

Sand the ends of the dowel after it's been cut. You don't want any little splintered wood pieces in your pressed powders!

Getting the right amount of jojoba oil to hold the pressed powders together and not be too oily is a little tricky. Too much jojoba oil, and the powder will stick to the dowel. Too little, and it won't hold the powder together. Here's what seems to work best:

1. After you've blended the makeup and added the ¼ teaspoon (1.2 milliliters) jojoba oil and the preservative, use a pipette to add 2 more drops jojoba oil. Blend for at least 1 minute.

2. Then using the same pipette, add 4 more drops jojoba oil, and grind the powders for another minute.

3. Spoon some of the powder into the jar, and using your dowel and a small hammer or something to tap on the top of the dowel, gently tap on the end of the dowel, pressing the powders into the jar.

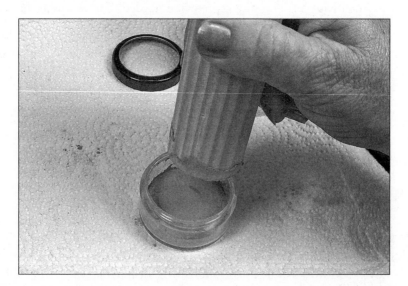

4. Add more powder, and repeat until the jar is full.

5. When the jar is just about full, add the last amount of powder. Then place a pressing ribbon or a small piece of fabric on top, and press to give your pressed powders a nice finish.

These powders will still break and crumble if they're carried loose in a purse, but they'll hold together well otherwise.

TKB Trading has special tools and ribbon for pressing your powders. These are inexpensive and easy to use. They also have a new liquid binder for pressing the powders. Check them out at tkbtrading.com.

Making Mineral Foundations

Now for the fun stuff! The first thing you want to choose is the type of coverage you want for your foundation. I have three types:

- Sheer

- Medium

- Maximum coverage

This base filler makes up the largest part of your foundation and is what you add the color grind to. The base filler is just a start, and you may want to add or omit ingredients later.

The base filler recipes yield 4 ounces (113.4 grams). That makes up 75 to 90 percent of your foundation recipe. If you don't want 4 ounces (113.4 grams) filler, just cut the amount for each ingredient in half and make 2 ounces (56.7 grams).

IN THE MIRROR

These recipes usually go over the 100 percent amount because we usually don't count the preservative and/or fragrance in formulations. I like to use Optiphen Plus preservative. It's paraben- and formaldehyde-free.

Here's what you need to make mineral foundations:

- Scale (one that weighs to the 100th is great)

- Face mask

- Latex gloves

- Waxed paper

- Small paper cups

- Coffee grinder or mortar and pestle

- 6-inch dowel rods the diameter of your containers (for making pressed powder) or TKB Trading pressing tools

- Zipper-lock bag or 30-gram shifter jar

Natural Sheer Base Filler

This almost-transparent base is the best for young skin that just needs a little color in the evening. This is also the filler base recipe we use for the bronzers. You can cut this in half or double it to make a larger amount. This recipe makes 4 ounces (113.4 grams) base filler.

French or rose talc	2.5 ounces (70.9 grams)
Titanium dioxide	.3 ounce (8.5 grams)
Silk mica or rice powder	.8 ounce (22.7 grams)
Magnesium stearate	.1 ounce (2.8 grams)
Zinc oxide	.3 ounce (8.5 grams)
Preservative	(see manufacturer's recommendation)

1. Put on your face mask and gloves, and put a piece of waxed paper over your work area.

2. Set your scale to grams, put a small cup on the scale, and push the tare button.

3. Weigh the first ingredient, and pour it into the grinder bowl or mortar.

4. Replace the cup on the scale, push the tare button again, and continue weighing all the ingredients except the preservative.

5. Put the grinder bowl on the grinder, and grind in short spurts for 1 minute. If you're using a mortar and pestle, hand-grind the powders for several minutes. What you should see is an intense skin-tone color.

6. Add the preservative, and grind again in short spurts for 2 minutes. If using a mortar and pestle, grind for 4 or 5 minutes.

7. Store the base filler in a zipper-lock bag or a clean jar until you're ready to mix it with a color grind.

Medium-Coverage Base Filler

This is a medium-coverage finish that offers a little more coverage than the sheer but not as much as the maximum. If you want, you can cut this recipe in half or double it to make a larger amount. This recipe makes 4 ounces (113.4 grams) base filler.

French or rose talc	2.1 ounces (59.5 grams)
Titanium dioxide	.8 ounce (22.7 grams)
Sericite mica	.6 ounce (17 grams)
Magnesium stearate	.1 ounce (2.8 grams)
Zinc oxide	.4 ounce (11.3 grams)
Preservative	(see manufacturer's recommendation)

Prepare as directed in the Natural Sheer Base Filler recipe.

Maximum-Coverage Base Filler

This base filler gives the best coverage for mature or acne-scarred skin. It's the one I use. If you like, you can cut this recipe in half or double it to make a larger amount. This recipe makes 4 ounces (113.4 grams) base filler.

French or rose talc	1.7 ounces (48.2 grams)
Titanium dioxide	.5 ounce (14.2 grams)
Sericite mica	.7 ounce (19.8 grams)
Silk mica	.5 ounce (14.2 grams)
Magnesium stearate	.2 ounce (5.7 grams)
Zinc oxide	.4 ounce (11.3 grams)
Preservative	(see manufacturer's recommendation)

Prepare as directed in the Natural Sheer Base Filler recipe.

IN THE MIRROR

All iron oxides and micas are synthetically made and duplicated exactly from the natural oxides and micas found in the earth. This is done so all the colorants are sterile and don't contain contaminants. The Food and Drug Administration lists these synthetic iron oxides and micas as color additives that are safe, so they don't have to be listed on the product label. However, lake dyes and FD&C colorants do have to be listed on labels even though they're approved for eyes, lips, face, or nails.

Making Color Grinds

These grinds are the second part of the foundation—the color part—and make up 10 to 25 percent of your foundation. It's best to use a coffee bean grinder for these (they're faster and better at grinding evenly), but you also can use a mortar and pestle.

When deciding on a color, choose one that best describes your skin tone. Here are some common ingredients you'll use:

- Titanium dioxide (white)
- Yellow oxide (mustard yellow)
- Red oxide (true red)
- Red oxide—blue shade (maroon red)
- Black oxide (very dark black)
- Brown oxide (reddish brown)
- Dark brown oxide (brown with black)
- Chromium green oxide (medium green, not teal)
- Ultramarine blue (bright blue)
- Ultramarine violet (medium purple/violet, for color corrector)
- French or rose talc (translucent white)
- Jojoba oil (clear or golden)

To make more foundation colors, you can blend any of these grinds with the filler base. You can also use these oxides to make your concealers and color correctors.

After you've made your basic blend (instructions follow), test it on your skin in natural light. Rub some of the foundation on the inside of your forearm, and hold it in direct sunlight. If the foundation isn't dark enough, go back and add a little more ivory color grind and grind again. Continue doing this until you have the correct color.

IN THE MIRROR

Between the fifteenth and nineteenth centuries, it was very fashionable to whiten your face. The whiter the face, the idea went, the wealthier the person was, and therefore didn't need to spend time outdoors doing chores. During that time, most women whitened their faces using a mixture of carbonate, hydroxide, and lead oxide. Yuck!

Here's what you need to make color grinds:

- Scale
- Coffee grinder or mortar and pestle
- Tiny scoops
- Small paper cups
- 3mm pipettes
- Face mask

- Latex gloves
- Paper towels
- Bottle of 3 percent alcohol
- 30-gram sifter jars
- Oxides
- 6-inch dowel rods
- Waxed paper

These recipes are all written in grams because of the tiny amounts used for many of the colors in creating each blend.

Ivory Color Grind

This is a light ivory blend with touches of yellow. To cut the yellow undertones, you can use the violet corrector under this foundation to give you a more neutral skin tone. This recipe makes about 1 ounce (28.4 grams) color grind.

French or rose talc	15.8 grams
Titanium dioxide	7.4 grams
Yellow oxide	4 grams
Red oxide	.4 gram
Brown oxide	.4 gram
Preservative	(see manufacturer's recommendation)

1. Put on your face mask and gloves, and put a piece of waxed paper over your work area.

2. Set your scale to grams, put a small cup on the scale, and push the tare button.

3. Weigh the first ingredient, and pour it into the grinder bowl or mortar.

4. Replace the cup on the scale, push the tare button again, and continue weighing all the ingredients except the preservative.

5. Put the grinder bowl on the grinder, and grind in short spurts for 1 minute. If you're using a mortar and pestle, hand-grind the powders for several minutes. What you should see is an intense skin-tone color.

6. Add the preservative and grind again in short spurts for 2 minutes. If using a mortar and pestle, grind for 4 or 5 minutes.

To make your foundation, you'll combine the color grinds and a base filler. This will make 1 ounce (28.4 grams) foundation. Package in a zipper-lock bag or a 30-gram sifter jar.

1. Put on your face mask and gloves, and put a piece of waxed paper over your work area.

2. Place a small paper cup on the scale, and push the tare button to zero out the weight of the cup. Weigh .8 ounce (22.7 grams) your choice of base filler. Pour it into the grinder bowl or mortar.

3. Place a clean paper cup on the scale and again push the tare button. Weigh .2 ounce (5.7 grams) color grind. Pour into grinder bowl or mortar.

4. If you're using a grinder, grind for 1 minute in short spurts. If you're using a mortar and pestle, hand-grind the powders for several minutes. Rub some of the foundation on the inside of your forearm and look at it in sunlight. Make adjustments by adding a little more color grind or base filler. Grind again. Check the color again in sunlight. Do this until your color is right for your skin tone. Be sure to make notes about how much extra grind or filler base you added so next time you won't have to do so much adjusting.

5. Add ¼ teaspoon (1.2 milliliters) jojoba oil, plus the extra drops, if desired, for pressing your foundation. Grind again as before.

6. Store unused color grind and base filler in jars or zipper-lock bags.

PRETTY POINTER

If you have an ivory skin tone that has pink tones, change the red oxide in this recipe to 0.6 gram and add 0.2 gram ultramarine blue.

Sand Tone Color Grind

This color grind is for light olive skin with yellow undertones. This recipe makes about 1 ounce (28.4 grams) color grind.

French or rose talc	15.4 grams
Titanium dioxide	6.3 grams
Yellow oxide	3.6 grams

Brown oxide	1.2 grams
Red oxide	.8 gram
Ultramarine blue	.4 gram
Black oxide	.3 gram
Preservative	(see manufacturer's recommendation)

Prepare as directed in the Ivory Color Grind recipe.

Gold Tone Color Grind

This is for light to medium olive skin tones with a gold undertone. This recipe makes about 1 ounce (28.4 grams) color grind.

French or rose talc	13.1 grams
Titanium dioxide	6.3 grams
Yellow oxide	7.9 grams
Brown oxide	.4 gram
Red oxide	.3 gram
Preservative	(see manufacturer's recommendation)

Prepare as directed in the Ivory Color Grind recipe.

Sun Deep Gold Color Grind

This grind is for darker-medium warm golden skin tones with a yellow undertone. This recipe makes about 1 ounce (28.4 grams) color grind.

French or rose talc	14.9 grams
Titanium dioxide	6.3 grams
Yellow oxide	5.3 grams
Red oxide	1.1 grams
Black oxide	.4 gram
Preservative	(see manufacturer's recommendation)

Prepare as directed in the Ivory Color Grind recipe.

Honey Russet Color Grind

This grind is for medium-warm skin tones with a red undertone. This recipe makes about 1 ounce (28.4 grams) color grind.

French or rose talc	12.4 grams
Titanium dioxide	6.3 grams
Yellow oxide	5.4 grams
Red oxide	3.9 grams
Black oxide	.4 gram
Preservative	(see manufacturer's recommendation)

Prepare as directed in the Ivory Color Grind recipe.

Olive Color Grind

This grind is for the deeper, neutral olive tones. This recipe makes about 1 ounce (28.4 grams) color grind.

French or rose talc	12.8 grams
Titanium dioxide	5.5 grams
Yellow oxide	5.5 grams
Red oxide—blue shade	1.2 grams
Red oxide	1.1 grams
Chromium green oxide	.6 gram
Black oxide	.5 gram
Brown oxide	.4 gram
Ultramarine blue	.4 gram
Preservative	(see manufacturer's recommendation)

Prepare as directed in the Ivory Color Grind recipe.

Rose Tones Color Grind

This grind is for the rosy tones. This recipe makes about 1 ounce (28.4 grams) color grind.

French or rose talc	13.8 grams
Titanium dioxide	7.8 grams

Yellow oxide	3.5 grams
Red oxide	1.9 grams
Red oxide—blue shade	.8 gram
Ultramarine blue	.5 gram
Preservative	(see manufacturer's recommendation)

Prepare as directed in the Ivory Color Grind recipe.

Bronze Color Grind

This grind is for medium- to deep-brown tones. This recipe makes about 1 ounce (28.4 grams) color grind.

French or rose talc	14.2 grams
Titanium dioxide	6.3 grams
Yellow oxide	5.8 grams
Red oxide	1.4 grams
Black oxide	.3 gram
Preservative	(see manufacturer's recommendation)

Prepare as directed in the Ivory Color Grind recipe.

Making Color Correctors

Many of us have too much red or yellow in our skin tones. For these skin tone problems, it's color correctors to the rescue. Simply apply these little wonders after you've applied your moisturizer and before your foundation. For the ruddy tone (red), use the green corrector, and for a sallow (yellow) skin tone, apply the violet color corrector. For dark circles under your eyes, use the yellow corrector. Use in problem areas or all over your face, and you'll really tell the difference.

Here's what you need to make color correctors:

- Coffee grinder or mortar and pestle
- 30-gram sifter jar
- Scale
- Paper cups
- 3mm pipettes
- 6-inch dowels the diameter of the jars

Green Color Corrector

Use this color corrector on red tones or red spots and blotches. This recipe makes 1 ounce (28.4 grams) color corrector.

French or rose talc	13.5 grams
Titanium dioxide	7.3 grams
Chromium green oxide	3.4 grams
Yellow oxide	4 grams
Jojoba oil	¼ teaspoon (1.2 milliliters)
Preservative	(see manufacturer's recommendation)

1. Put on your face mask and gloves, and put a piece of waxed paper over your work area.

2. Set your scale to grams, put one of the small cups on the scale, and push the tare button. Weigh the first powder, and pour it into the grinder bowl or mortar.

3. Replace the cup on the scale, push the tare button, and continue until you've weighed all the ingredients except the jojoba oil and preservative.

4. Place in the grinder and grind in short spurts for 1 minute. If you're using a mortar and pestle, hand-grind the powders for several minutes.

5. Add the jojoba oil and preservative. Grind again in short spurts for 2 minutes. If you're using a mortar and pestle, grind for 4 or 5 minutes.

6. Fill a sterile 30-gram sifter jar.

Violet Color Corrector

Use this color corrector on yellow tones. This recipe makes 1 ounce (28.4 grams) color corrector.

French or rose talc	17 grams
Titanium dioxide	6 grams
Ultramarine violet	5.4 grams

| Jojoba oil | ¼ teaspoon (1.2 milliliters) |
| Preservative | (see manufacturer's recommendation) |

Prepare as directed in the Green Color Corrector recipe.

Yellow Color Corrector

Use this color corrector on blue areas such as dark circles under eyes. This recipe makes 1 ounce (28.4 grams) color corrector.

French or rose talc	16.1 grams
Titanium dioxide	8.1 grams
Yellow oxide	4.1 grams
Jojoba oil	¼ teaspoon (1.2 milliliters)
Preservative	(see manufacturer's recommendation)

Prepare as directed in the Green Color Corrector recipe.

Making Concealer

We all need a little extra coverage once in a while and would rather not look like we have plaster on our faces. For these times and other special small areas, we use a concealer. Concealer is very simple to make and just as simple to use. After you've used your moisturizer, apply the concealer before you put on your foundation. You can double these recipes as many times as you want to make the batch size you want.

Here's what you need to make concealer:

- Scale

- Paper cups

- Coffee grinder or mortar and pestle

- 30-gram sifter jar

- 6-inch dowels the diameter of the jar

Concealer

You can make your own personalized concealer from the color grind you've matched to your skin tone earlier in this chapter and with the same base filler. Mix these 50–50 with the jojoba oil. This recipe makes 1 ounce (28.4 grams) concealer.

Base filler	14.2 grams
Color grind	14.2 grams
Jojoba oil	¼ teaspoon (1.2 milliliters)

1. Put on your face mask and gloves, and put a piece of waxed paper over your work area.

2. Weigh and place all ingredients in a grinder or mortar, and blend very well.

3. Store concealer in a 30-gram sifter jar. Apply to face, using a makeup brush, after your moisturizer and before your foundation. Use your makeup brush to blend the concealer well. You don't want any makeup lines or blotches.

> **PRETTY POINTER**
>
> If you feel you need a little more coverage, you can apply more concealer over your foundation. You can also use the base filler that has more coverage, if you desire.

The Least You Need to Know

- Look at your skin in the sunlight and decide which color grind best describes your skin tone. Roll up your sleeves and get started!

- Making your own mineral makeup is doable with our easy-to-follow step-by-step instructions.

- Once you try mineral makeup, you'll never go back to any other kind. It feels like you have nothing on your face and looks so natural, too!

Blushes and Bronzers

In This Chapter

- Blushes for that beautiful, healthy look
- Bronzers for a healthy glow—without all the other makeup

Don't you love how your face looks (and how you feel!) when you have a little color in your cheeks? In this chapter, we share several color grinds for blushes and bronzers to give you that little extra something.

And here's a bonus: they're easier to make than the foundations in Chapter 8! If you worked through Chapter 8, you'll be a step ahead here because you blend blushes and bronzers very similarly to how you blended the foundations.

The Basics of Making Blush

To help you choose the right blush for your skin tone, think what color your skin turns when you are flushed or embarrassed. Blushing is when the blood rushes to the surface of the skin. Your blush, therefore, should reflect those color tones for a more natural look. Someone with fair skin blushes pink. They do not blush plum.

Here's what you need to make blush:

- TKB Trading Matte Texture Base
- Set of 5 TKB stainless-steel measuring spoons (Tad, Dash, Pinch, Smidgen, and Drop sizes)
- Coffee grinder or mortar and pestle
- Scale
- 3mm pipettes
- 30-gram sifter jars

- Alcohol or 3 percent hydrogen peroxide

- Several small paper cups

- Face mask

- Latex gloves

- Paper towels

- Waxed paper

- 6-inch dowel rods the diameter of the jars (for making pressed powder)

IN THE MIRROR

Besides using a scale for weighing the colorants, I also frequently use a set of five stainless-steel measuring spoons (not the set of three) sold at TKB Trading. These little measuring spoons are very small and called Tad, Dash, Pinch, Smidgen, and Drop. Sometimes you only need a Pinch or a Dash or a Smidgen, and the scale just can't weigh that tiny amount. Also, it's hard to weigh an odd amount, such as .24 grams oxide. Using the Pinch spoon, you can do it easily! When you see *Tad, Dash, Pinch, Smidgen,* and *Drop* in the ingredient lists, please note that these are referring to these measuring spoons. (See Appendix D for ordering info.)

As mentioned earlier, cleanliness is very important when it comes to making beauty products. Be sure you wash your jars and utensils in hot, soapy water and let air-dry. Then swish alcohol in the containers, lids, sifters, and bowl of the grinder or mortar. Let them air-dry again. Put the jar pieces in zipper-lock bags until you're ready to fill them.

Clean your workspace with vinegar or 3 percent hydrogen peroxide, and cover your work surface with waxed paper. Keep a bottle of alcohol and a roll of paper towels handy for quick wipes or cleanups. These oxides and micas can be messy!

If you're making pressed blushes and bronzers, you'll need a tamping rod (see Chapter 8).

Making Color Grinds for Blushes

You will want to pick a color grind that goes with your skin tone. If you don't know what color your cheeks are when you're flushed, you can pinch and gently slap them until the blood comes to the surface. Don't do this to the point of causing bruises! Do it just enough so you can see the color tone. Matching that color for your blush makes the most becoming and natural look on you.

I buy all my oxides and micas from TKB Trading (see Appendix D) and have used the exact name of each mica and oxide so you'll know which one to use to get the exact color for these grinds. If there is too much "sparkle" in your color grind, just add a little more of the TKB Matte Texture Base, and that should do the trick. Some micas have more sparkle than others.

Each of the following recipes makes about 1 ounce (28.4 grams) blush and will fill a 30-gram sifter jar. If you press the blush, you may want to double the recipe so it fills the jar completely. There will be a little left over after pressing.

SAFETY FIRST

It's very important to use an across-the-board preservative in these products, one that kills germs and bacteria. I recommend Optiphen Plus. It's paraben- and formaldehyde-free. (See Appendix E for more on preservatives.)

Pink Tones

These are best suited for those whose skin tone matches the Ivory Color Grind in Chapter 8, and they're great blushes for young teens.

Sweet Valentine Blush

A soft, medium true pink. This blush goes on light and will add just a healthy touch of pink to the cheeks. It's best suited for very fair skin. This recipe makes 1 ounce (28.4 grams).

Titanium dioxide	.05 ounce (1.4 grams)
Magnesium Violet	.3 ounce (8.5 grams)
Yellow oxide	.08 ounce (2.3 grams)
Red oxide	2 Tads
Ultramarine Blue	1 Tad
French or rose talc	.25 ounce (7.1 grams)
Magnesium stearate	.2 ounce (5.7 grams)
Rice powder or silk mica	.1 ounce (2.8 grams)
Jojoba oil	.035 ounce (1 gram; 1 milliliter)
Preservative	(see manufacturer's recommendation)

1. Put on your face mask and gloves, and put a piece of waxed paper over your work area.

2. Set your scale to grams or ounces, place a small cup or bowl on the scale, and push the tare button. This zeroes out the weight of the container.

3. Weigh the first oxide or mica. Transfer it to your coffee grinder or mortar. Put the cup or bowl back on the scale, and again push the tare button. Continue weighing each colorant in the recipe until you have each one transferred and ready to grind.

4. Grind the colorants for several seconds. Check your color by rubbing a little of the blend on the back of your hand.

5. Add the jojoba oil and the preservative to the coffee grinder or mortar, and grind for 1 minute. Shake the bowl around to redistribute the powder, and grind for another minute. If you're making pressed blush, add 6 to 10 extra drops jojoba oil (using the 3mm pipette), and grind again.

6. Fill your 30-gram sifter jar by spooning in a little powder at a time. If you're pressing the powder, pack it in using the 6-inch dowel tamper. Spoon half the powder into the jar, and press down with the dowel, using something to tap on the top of the dowel to press the powder tight. Fill the jar with the rest of the powder and repeat tapping with the dowel. Alternatively, you can leave the powder loose and just use a spoon to fill the sifter jar.

7. Place the lid on the jar, and store it until you're ready to use.

SAFETY FIRST

Working with micas and oxides can be very messy. Because they're so lightweight, they easily float in the air, and they can end up in your lungs if you're not careful. To avoid this, wear a face mask while working with the micas and oxides. Also, cover your workspace with a piece of waxed paper to make cleanup easier. They may also end up on your clothes, so wear an old T-shirt while working.

Sweetly Innocent Blush

A medium true pink with warm undertones. This blush is best suited for those with medium-fair skin that has a touch of yellow tone. This recipe makes about 1 ounce (28.4 grams).

Be My Valentine mica	.3 ounce (8.5 grams)
Cloisonne Red mica	.15 ounce (4.3 grams)
Rouge Flambe Red mica	1 Tad
French or rose talc	.35 ounce (9.9 grams)

Magnesium stearate	.1 ounce (2.8 grams)
Rice powder or silk mica	.05 ounce (1.4 grams)
Jojoba oil	.035 ounce (1 gram; 1 milliliter)
Preservative	(see manufacturer's recommendation)

Prepare as directed in the Sweet Valentine Blush recipe.

Sweetheart Pink Blush

A soft, true pink. This blush isn't as light as the Sweet Valentine Blush, but it's still soft. It's best suited for fair skin with warm undertones. This recipe makes 1.2 ounces (34 grams).

Blush Beige mica	.3 ounce (8.5 grams)
Tibetan Ochre mica	.15 ounce (4.3 grams)
Cotton Candy mica	.3 ounce (8.5 grams)
TKB Trading Matte Texture Base	.05 ounce (1.4 grams)
French or rose talc	.15 ounce (4.3 grams)
Magnesium stearate	.125 ounce (3.5 grams)
Rice powder or silk mica	.05 ounce (1.4 grams)
Jojoba oil	.035 ounce (1 gram; 1 milliliter)
Preservative	(see manufacturer's recommendation)

Prepare as directed in the Sweet Valentine Blush recipe.

Rosy Tones

No matter what undertones your skin has, you'll find a rosy tone blush that will work for you. These colors work for daytime, office wear, and even evening wear. They're the most natural-looking blushes for most skin tones and give you a healthy glow. Remember, when you really blush, you don't blush orange or purple.

Pink Rose Blush

A beautiful rosy pink. This blush has an intense rosy color. It's very suitable for light to medium skin tones. This recipe makes 1 ounce (28.4 grams).

Ultramarine Pink mica	.05 ounce (1.4 grams)
Magnesium Violet mica	.275 ounce (7.8 grams)
Titanium dioxide	.05 ounce (1.4 grams)

Red oxide	1 Pinch
French or rose talc	.4 ounce (11.3 grams)
Magnesium stearate	.1 ounce (2.8 grams)
Rice powder or silk mica	.05 ounce (1.4 grams)
Jojoba oil	.035 ounce (1 gram; 1 milliliter)
Preservative	(see manufacturer's recommendation)

Prepare as directed in the Sweet Valentine Blush recipe.

Soft Rose Blush

A soft rose with neutral tones. This blush has a splash more of color that will brighten your whole face. It's best suited for any light to medium skin tone and any type undertone. This recipe makes 1 ounce (28.4 grams).

Sparkling Rose mica	0.3 ounce (8.5 grams)
TKB Trading Matte Texture Base	.2 ounce (5.7 grams)
Red #40	.05 ounce (1.4 grams)
Hot Momma mica	.07 ounce (2 grams)
French or rose talc	.2 ounce (5.7 grams)
Magnesium stearate	.12 ounce (3.4 grams)
Rice powder or silk mica	.05 ounce (1.4 grams)
Jojoba oil	.035 ounce (1 gram; 1 milliliter)
Preservative	(see manufacturer's recommendation)

Prepare as directed in the Sweet Valentine Blush recipe.

Hot House Rose Blush

A medium-warm-tone rose. This blush will have you kicking up your heels and looking great! It's perfect for warm skin tones. This recipe makes just over 1 ounce (30 grams).

Hot Momma mica	.35 ounce (9.9 grams)
TKB Trading Matte Texture Base	.35 ounce (9.9 grams)
French or rose talc	.2 ounce (5.7 grams)
Magnesium stearate	.1 ounce (2.8 grams)
Rice powder or silk mica	.05 ounce (1.4 grams)

| Jojoba oil | .035 ounce (1 gram; 1 milliliter) |
| Preservative | (see manufacturer's recommendation) |

Prepare as directed in the Sweet Valentine Blush recipe.

Trinity Blush

A soft, neutral rose. This blush contains just enough color for day wear without looking overly made up. It works well for both warm and cool skin tones. This recipe makes just under 1 ounce (24 grams).

Sparkling Rose mica	.2 ounce (5.7 grams)
Colorona Bordeaux mica	.2 ounce (5.7 grams)
Red #40	2 Tads
TKB Trading Matte Texture Base	.2 ounce (5.7 grams)
French or rose talc	.2 ounce (5.7 grams)
Magnesium stearate	.1 ounce (2.8 grams)
Rice powder or silk mica	.05 ounce (1.4 grams)
Jojoba oil	.035 ounce (1 gram; 1 milliliter)
Preservative	(see manufacturer's recommendation)

Prepare as directed in the Sweet Valentine Blush recipe.

Deep Red Tones

When we blush, red is the main color our cheeks turn. For evening-wear makeup, red is the color. There's a red for each complexion type in this section. Choose the one that suits you best.

Wine and Roses Blush

A deep wine blush. This blush is best suited for medium to dark complexions. It has a slight blue undertone and is perfect for those who look best in cool-tone colors. This recipe makes 1 ounce (28.4 grams).

Titanium dioxide	.125 ounce (3.5 grams)
Magnesium Violet mica	.25 ounce (7.1 grams)
Red oxide	.075 ounce (2.1 grams)
Red oxide—blue shade	1 Tad

French or rose talc	.25 ounce (7.1 grams)
Magnesium stearate	.17 ounce (4.8 grams)
Rice powder or silk mica	.08 ounce (2.3 grams)
Jojoba oil	.035 ounce (1 gram; 1 milliliter)
Preservative	(see manufacturer's recommendation)

Prepare as directed in the Sweet Valentine Blush recipe.

Deep Rosy Red Blush

A deep rose so deep it's almost a red. This blush gives you a healthy and beautiful glow. It's best suited for those with medium to dark cool complexions. This recipe makes 1 ounce (28.4 grams).

Red oxide	.04 ounce (1.1 grams)
Magnesium Violet mica	.15 ounce (4.3 grams)
TKB Trading Matte Texture Base	.3 ounce (8.5 grams)
Sparkling Rose mica	.15 ounce (4.3 grams)
French or rose talc	.175 ounce (5 grams)
Magnesium stearate	.12 ounce (3.4 grams)
Rice powder or silk mica	.06 ounce (1.7 grams)
Jojoba oil	.035 ounce (1 gram; 1 milliliter)
Preservative	(see manufacturer's recommendation)

Prepare as directed in the Sweet Valentine Blush recipe.

Deeply Red Blush

A dark warm red. This blush is best suited for darker warm complexions. This recipe makes just over 1 ounce (30 grams).

Red oxide	.1 ounce (2.8 grams)
Colorona Bordeaux mica	.2 ounce (5.7 grams)
TKB Trading Matte Texture Base	.4 ounce (11.3 grams)
French or rose talc	.2 ounce (5.7 grams)
Magnesium stearate	.1 ounce (2.8 grams)
Rice powder or silk mica	.05 ounce (1.4 grams)

Jojoba oil	.035 ounce (1 gram; 1 milliliter)
Preservative	(see manufacturer's recommendation)

Prepare as directed in the Sweet Valentine Blush recipe.

Lucille Blush

A true red. This blush is bright! A little goes a long way. It's well suited for medium complexions that have warm tones. This recipe makes just over 1 ounce (31 grams).

Carmine	.15 ounce (4.3 grams)
Red #40	.075 ounce (2.1 grams)
Red oxide	.1 ounce (2.8 grams)
Queen Kathryn mica	1 Tad plus 1 Pinch
TKB Trading Matte Texture Base	.4 ounce (11.3 grams)
French or rose talc	.2 ounce (5.7 grams)
Magnesium stearate	.1 ounce (2.8 grams)
Rice powder or silk mica	.05 ounce (1.4 grams)
Jojoba oil	.035 ounce (1 gram; 1 milliliter)
Preservative	(see manufacturer's recommendation)

Prepare as directed in the Sweet Valentine Blush recipe.

Peach Tones

We all love the soft, peach-tone blushes. They work so well with so many complexions and hair colors. Here you'll find several to choose from. We know you'll find at least one here to love.

Peaches and Apricot Blush

A nice peach/apricot blush. This blush is well suited for light to medium skin tones that have warm undertones. This recipe makes 1 ounce (28.4 grams).

Magnesium Violet mica	.3 ounce (8.5 grams)
Yellow oxide	.17 ounce (4.8 grams)
Orange oxide	.15 ounce (4.3 grams)
Red oxide	.08 ounce (2.3 grams)
Brown oxide	1 Tad plus 1 Smidgen

French or rose talc	.1 ounce (2.8 grams)
Magnesium stearate	.1 ounce (2.8 grams)
Titanium dioxide	.1 ounce (2.8 grams)
Jojoba oil	.035 ounce (1 gram; 1 milliliter)
Preservative	(see manufacturer's recommendation)

Prepare as directed in the Sweet Valentine Blush recipe.

Romance Blush

A beautiful medium peach tone. This blush is perfect for medium-light complexions with warm tones. This recipe makes just over 1 ounce (29 grams).

Butter Yellow mica	.15 ounce (4.3 grams)
Scarlet O'Hara mica	.15 ounce (4.3 grams)
Red oxide	.05 ounce (1.4 grams)
Yellow oxide	1 Pinch
Titanium dioxide	.15 ounce (4.3 grams)
French or rose talc	.25 ounce (7.1 grams)
Magnesium stearate	.15 ounce (4.3 grams)
Rice powder or silk mica	.1 ounce (2.8 grams)
Jojoba oil	.035 ounce (1 gram; 1 milliliter)
Preservative	(see manufacturer's recommendation)

Prepare as directed in the Sweet Valentine Blush recipe.

Lightly Dusted Peach Blush

A soft apricot and peach blush with a hint of cinnamon. Have a light tan? This blush would be perfect! This recipe makes just over 1 ounce (30 grams).

Sparkling Rose mica	.1 ounce (2.8 grams)
Pink Coral mica	.2 ounce (5.7 grams)
Apricot mica	.2 ounce (5.7 grams)
Antique Copper mica	.08 ounce (2.1 grams)
TKB Trading Matte Texture Base	.05 ounce (1.4 grams)
French or rose talc	.25 ounce (7.1 grams)
Magnesium stearate	.08 ounce (2.3 grams)

Rice powder or silk mica	.075 ounce (2.1 grams)
Jojoba oil	.035 ounce (1 gram; 1 milliliter)
Preservative	(see manufacturer's recommendation)

Prepare as directed in the Sweet Valentine Blush recipe.

Plum Tones

No one blushes a plum color, but for those with darker complexions, the plum blushes can be gorgeous! If you've ever had your colors done, you know colors are divided into two groups: warm and cool. If you look better in gold, you're a warm tone; if you look better in silver, you're a cool tone. To wear these colors, you have to have a darker complexion with a cool tone. Remember, plum has both red and blues, making it a cool color.

Sweet Plum Blush

A medium plum with a hint of pink undertone. This blush is not for blondes or those with fair complexions. This recipe makes 1 ounce (28.4 grams).

Sparkling Rose mica	.2 ounce (5.7 grams)
Manganese Violet	.2 ounce (5.7 grams)
Oriental Beige mica	.2 ounce (5.7 grams)
French or rose talc	.2 ounce (5.7 grams)
Magnesium stearate	.1 ounce (2.8 grams)
Rice powder or silk mica	.05 ounce (1.4 grams)
Jojoba oil	.035 ounce (1 gram; 1 milliliter)
Preservative	(see manufacturer's recommendation)

Prepare as directed in the Sweet Valentine Blush recipe.

Plum 'N' Berries Blush

A deep plum with red undertones. This blush is dramatic! This recipe makes 1 ounce (28.4 grams).

Manganese Violet mica	.2 ounce (5.7 grams)
Antique Copper mica	.2 ounce (5.7 grams)
Colorona Russet mica	3 Tads plus 1 Pinch

French or rose talc	.3 ounce (8.5 grams)
Magnesium stearate	.15 ounce (4.3 grams)
Rice powder or silk mica	.1 ounce (2.8 grams)
Jojoba oil	.035 ounce (1 gram; 1 milliliter)
Preservative	(see manufacturer's recommendation)

Prepare as directed in the Sweet Valentine Blush recipe.

Brown-Cinnamon Tones

This is another blush group that works well with so many different complexions and hair colors. This group is best suited for the warm tones, from fair to dark complexions.

My Azure Blush

A medium cinnamon tone with a touch of gold and red undertones. You can use this grind for lipstick, too! Just use the first 3 ingredients. This recipe makes just under 1 ounce (20 grams).

Cote'd Azure mica	.2 ounce (5.7 grams)
Swiss Chocolate mica	.1 ounce (2.8 grams)
Red oxide	1 Drop
French or rose talc	.215 ounce (6.1 grams)
Magnesium stearate	.075 ounce (2.1 grams)
Sericite mica	.05 ounce (1.4 grams)
Rice powder or silk mica	.056 ounce (1.6 grams)
Jojoba oil	.035 ounce (1 gram; 1 milliliter)
Preservative	(see manufacturer's recommendation)

Prepare as directed in the Sweet Valentine Blush recipe.

Cinnamon-Apple Blush

A soft cinnamon with red undertones. This blush is soft enough for fair skin and deep enough for darker complexions, too. This recipe makes 1.4 ounces (39.7 grams).

Queen Kathryn mica	.6 ounce (17 grams)
Antique Copper mica	.4 ounce (11.3 grams)

French or rose talc	.2 ounce (5.7 grams)
Magnesium stearate	.1 ounce (2.8 grams)
Rice powder or silk mica	.07 ounce (2 grams)
Jojoba oil	.035 ounce (1 gram; 1 milliliter)
Preservative	(see manufacturer's recommendation)

Prepare as directed in the Sweet Valentine Blush recipe.

Tibetan Sunset Blush

A dark cinnamon with red undertones. This deep blush is best suited for darker complexions. It's not suitable for fair to medium skin tones. It does make a beautiful shade of lipstick using the first three ingredients! This recipe makes just under 1 ounce (28 grams).

Tibetan Ochre mica	.35 ounce (9.9 grams)
Swiss Chocolate mica	.35 ounce (9.9 grams)
Queen Kathryn mica	3 Tads
French or rose talc	.1 ounce (2.8 grams)
Magnesium stearate	.05 ounce (1.4 grams)
Rice powder or silk mica	.05 ounce (1.4 grams)
Jojoba oil	.035 ounce (1 gram; 1 milliliter)
Preservative	(see manufacturer's recommendation)

Prepare as directed in the Sweet Valentine Blush recipe.

IN THE MIRROR

Who were the first people to use blush? The ancient Egyptians. All through history, having a redness to the cheeks was thought to be beautiful and a sign of good health and youth. Just about anything that would stain the cheeks was used. In ancient Greece, for example, mulberries were used as a blush.

Making Bronzers

For the times you don't want to take the time to fully put on makeup yet you want to still look nice (and not like the walking dead!), a good bronzer is the perfect solution. For young ladies, a good bronzer is all you need to add just the right amount of even color to brighten the face. If you feel the bronzer is too shiny, you can add more

TKB Trading Matte Texture Base to help tone down the sparkle. Micas are sparkly, so adjust them to your liking. Use Chapter 8's Natural Sheer Base Filler recipe to blend with the following color grinds.

Please weigh your micas and oxides carefully and as exactly as you possibly can.

Here's what you need to make bronzers:

- Set of 5 TKB stainless-steel measuring spoons (Tad, Dash, Pinch, Smidgen, and Drop sizes)
- Coffee grinder or mortar and pestle
- Scale
- Sandwich size or smaller zipper-lock bags
- Small scoops
- 3mm pipettes
- 30-gram sifter jars
- Alcohol or 3 percent hydrogen peroxide
- Small paper cups
- Face mask
- Latex gloves
- Paper towels
- Waxed paper
- 6-inch dowels the diameter of the containers (for making pressed powder)

Base Filler for Bronzers

Using a translucent powder, bronzers add a little more color to your skin—a healthy glow—when you don't want to wear makeup. Bronzers are made in two parts: the base filler (the white powder) and the color grind. Grind them together with a little jojoba oil, and you have a bronzer. Should you feel that you would like a little more coverage, you can always use one of the other base fillers, cutting the recipe in half, for foundations in Chapter 8. You can always add a little more of the grind for more color. This recipe makes 2 ounces (56.7 grams) of base filler, giving you extra for making adjustments in your bronzer.

French or rose talc	1.2 ounces (34 grams)
Rice powder	.5 ounce (14.2 grams)

Sericite mica	.2 ounce (5.7 grams)
Mica spheres	.1 ounce (2.8 grams)
Jojoba oil	.035 ounce (1 gram; 1 milliliter)
Preservative	(see manufacturer's recommendation)

1. Place a cup or bowl on the scale, and push the tare button to zero out the weight of the container. Weigh the talc and pour it into the grinder bowl or mortar. Return the cup or bowl to the scale and push the tare button again and weigh the next ingredient. Continue until you have all the ingredients weighed and in the grinder bowl or mortar.

2. If you're using a coffee grinder, grind the ingredients for 2 minutes. If you're using a mortar and pestle, hand-grind for at least 4 minutes.

3. Store in a zipper-lock bag until ready to use.

> **PRETTY POINTER**
>
> If you want a bronzer without so much sparkle, you'll have to make a few adjustments to the base filler. Start by adding .2 ounce (5.7 grams) titanium dioxide or kaolin clay, and decrease the talc to 1 ounce (28.4 grams). For ladies with darker complexions who want less sparkle, add .2 ounce (5.7 grams) Coconut Crush mica.

Very Light Bronzer Color Grind

This color grind is for the lightest skin tone; it adds just a tiny touch of color. This recipe makes enough color grind to add to .8 ounce (22.7 grams) base filler to fill 1 (30-gram) sifter jar.

Base Filler for Bronzers	.8 ounce (22.7 grams)
Bronze Fine mica	.085 ounce (2.4 grams; 2.4 milliliters)
Gold Fine mica	.018 ounce (.5 gram; .5 milliliter)
TKB Trading Matte Texture Base	.023 ounce (.7 gram; .7 milliliter)
Preservative	(see manufacturer's recommendation)

1. Put on your face mask and gloves, and put a piece of waxed paper over your work area.

2. Place a cup on the scale and push the tare button. Weigh the base filler. Transfer it to your coffee grinder or mortar. Measure the micas, and add them to the base filler.

3. Grind the base filler and the micas together for 1 minute in short spurts. Test color by rubbing some on the inside of your forearm and going out in the sunlight. Make any adjustments needed.

4. Add the preservative. Grind for 2 minutes if using a coffee grinder or 4 or 5 minutes if you're using a mortar and pestle. You want to be sure the preservative is well distributed throughout the powder.

5. Fill a sterilized, 30-gram sifter jar and store the remainder in a zipper-lock bag.

Medium-Light Bronzer Color Grind

A little more color but still a light shade and good for those with a medium-light complexion. This recipe makes enough color grind to add to .8 ounce (22.7 grams) base filler to fill 1 (30-gram) sifter jar.

Base Filler for Bronzers	.8 ounce (22.7 grams)
Bronze fine mica	.173 ounce (4.9 grams; 4.9 milliliters)
Gold fine mica	.018 ounce (.5 gram; .5 milliliter)
TKB Trading Matte Texture Base	.023 ounce (.7 gram; .7 milliliter)
Preservative	(see manufacturer's recommendation)

Prepare as directed in the Very Light Bronzer Color Grind recipe.

Medium Bronzer Color Grind

This color grind is suitable for light olive and beige skin tones. This recipe makes enough color grind to add to .8 ounce (22.7 grams) base filler to fill 1 (30-gram) sifter jar.

Base Filler for Bronzers	.8 ounce (22.7 grams)
Bronze Fine mica	.173 ounce (4.9 grams; 4.9 milliliters)
Gold Fine mica	.018 ounce (.5 gram; .5 milliliter)
Australian Umber mica	.18 ounce (5.1 grams; 5.1 milliliters)
TKB Trading Matte Texture Base	.023 ounce (.7 gram; .7 milliliter)
Preservative	(see manufacturer's recommendation)

Prepare as directed in the Very Light Bronzer Color Grind recipe.

Dark Bronzer Color Grind

Even if you do have a deep tan, you may still want to add a little "glow." This is the blend for you. This recipe makes enough color grind to add to .8 ounce (22.7 grams) base filler to fill 1 (30-gram) sifter jar.

Base Filler for Bronzers	.8 ounce (22.7 grams)
Bronze Fine mica	.173 ounce (4.9 grams; 4.9 milliliters)
Gold Fine mica	.018 ounce (.5 gram; .5 milliliter)
Australian Umber mica	.225 ounce (6.4 grams; 6.4 milliliters)
Umber mica	.018 ounce (.5 gram; .5 milliliter)
TKB Trading Matte Texture Base	.023 ounce (.7 gram; .7 milliliter)
Preservative	(see manufacturer's recommendation)

Prepare as directed in the Very Light Bronzer Color Grind recipe.

Even Darker Bronzer Color Grind

The deepest bronzer color, suitable for the darker complexions. This recipe makes enough color grind to add to .8 ounce (22.7 grams) base filler to fill 1 (30-gram) sifter jar.

Base Filler for Bronzers	.8 ounce (22.7 grams)
Bronze Fine mica	.173 ounce (4.9 grams; 4.9 milliliters)
Gold Fine mica	.018 ounce (.5 gram; .5 milliliter)
Australian Umber mica	.18 ounce (5.1 grams; 5.1 milliliters)
Dark Brown oxide	.21 ounce (6 grams; 6 milliliters)
Swiss Chocolate mica	.22 ounce (6.2 grams; 6.2 milliliters)
TKB Trading Matte Texture Base	.087 ounce (2.5 grams; 2.5 milliliters)
Preservative	(see manufacturer's recommendation)

Prepare as directed in the Very Light Bronzer Color Grind recipe.

The Least You Need to Know

- It's a lot easier to make blush than you might have thought. Find your very own perfect blush in this chapter.
- When you just want a little something, bronzers offer a touch of extra color and shimmer.
- Micas and oxides are fun to work with, but they are messy, too. Wear old clothes while making your mineral makeup.

For the Eyes

In This Chapter

- Easy-to-make eye shadow grinds
- DIY all-natural eyeliner
- Make your own natural, chemical-free mascara

This is my favorite chapter, the one I enjoyed writing the most. I was able to let go and be very creative with the shadow blends. My granddaughter and her friends put in their 2 cents as to what's "in" these days. (Funny thing: some of the "in" colors and techniques they're doing now were popular when I was a teen in the 1960s! I had fun remembering the past and making some of the colors Twiggy made so popular!)

According to my daughter and granddaughter, the double line eyeliner is coming back. This is where you make a wider line with white eyeliner and then make a thinner line close to the eyelashes with black liner. So very 1960s! If they started drawing little lashes under the bottom lashes, the look would be complete. Of course I had to show my granddaughter how to do this just in case that comes back, too.

The Basics of Making Eye Shadows

Eye shadows aren't difficult to make. By using the basic color wheel, you can create all the eye shadow colors you could ever want. Let these grinds get you started on creating your own eye shadow colors. Hundreds of micas, or colorants, are available to choose from, you'll have lots of fun experimenting to come up with new shades.

I buy all my micas online from TKB Trading (see Appendix D) and have listed all the micas in the following recipes by name so you can easily find them if you want to make these exact blends. When you're ready to start creating your own grinds, I hope what I've given you here will serve as a good guide and encourage your imagination.

You can blend the micas with just other micas and have a beautiful resulting color, but you can also have some fun by creating more color-intense shadows. To achieve this look, simply add a little oxide or TKB Trading Purely Matte Texture Base for Eyes to the mica.

You apply mica eye shadow a little differently from how you apply commercial eye shadow. Try using a brush if you want a less-intense color. Use a sponge-tip applicator for a heavier and more intense look.

IN THE MIRROR

The Maybelline Company was created by T. L. Williams. He made the first "modern" mascara by mixing coal dust and Vaseline Petroleum Jelly. The name Maybelline came from combining Mr. Williams' sister's name, Maybel, and Vaseline.

Here's what you need to make eye shadows:

- Coffee grinder or mortar and pestle
- Scales
- Small scoops
- 3mm pipettes
- Waxed paper
- Set of 5 TKB stainless-steel measuring spoons (Tad, Dash, Pinch, Smidgen, and Drop sizes)
- Small paper cups or small lightweight bowls
- 10-gram sifter jars
- Alcohol
- Paper towels
- Face mask
- Latex gloves
- 6-inch dowels the diameter of the jars (for making pressed eye shadows) or TKB's pressing tools

PRETTY POINTER

To help prevent your eye shadow from creasing on your eyelids, try adding a few drops of hydrogenated polyisbutene in the final grinding.

As mentioned in other chapters, be sure your 10-milliliter sifter jars and other supplies as well as your workspace are all clean and sanitized. And always wash your hands thoroughly before you begin.

Making Eye Shadow Color Grinds

We begin by making shadow grinds that are about 10 to 15 grams each—just enough to fill the 10-gram sifter jars. For pressed shadow, double the recipe so you have enough to completely fill the jar.

If you have brown eyes, the warm colors will look sensational on you, as will golds and bronzes. Blue eyes sparkle with blues, warm browns, bronzes, and lavenders. Green eyes pop with purples as well as with roses, greens, and golds. If you have hazel eyes, you can't go wrong with browns, golds, coppers, greens, purples, plums, and sables.

You can also use these color grinds to make eyeliner pencils and color your mascara. Press these shadows, and you can rub them gently with a damp eyeliner brush and line your eyes. And you can always increase the amount you make by doubling the recipes as many times as you need to. Store the extra grind in zipper-lock bags.

PRETTY POINTER

I recommend using Optiphen Plus as your preservative. It's paraben- and formaldehyde-free. You wouldn't want to use a preservative that contained those chemicals on or around your eyes! I use a 3mm pipette to add 2 drops to the 10- to 15-gram eye shadow grinds.

Here is when you need the 5 TKB stainless-steel measuring spoons. Most scales won't weigh the tiny amounts of micas and oxides used in the following recipes. These little measuring spoons do the trick and are easy to use.

Highlighters

These light and creamy colors are perfect for under the eyebrow. Highlighters are always a light shade to draw attention to the shape of your eye and open up your eye.

Creamy White Eye Shadow

A very light shadow with a slight yellow or creamy color. This recipe makes enough grind to fill a 10-gram sifter jar.

Titanium dioxide	.05 ounce (1.4 grams)
Butter Yellow mica	.3 ounce (8.5 grams)
Bismuth Oxychloride Diamond Sheen	.05 ounce (1.4 grams)
Jojoba oil	⅛ teaspoon (.6 milliliter)
Preservative	2 drops

1. Place a piece of waxed paper on your counter in front of you. Set your scale to grams or ounces. Place a small paper cup on the scale, and push the tare button to zero out the weight of the cup.

2. Weigh the first oxide or mica. Transfer it to the coffee grinder or mortar. Put the cup back on the scale, and again push the tare button. Continue weighing each colorant until you have all transferred and ready to grind.

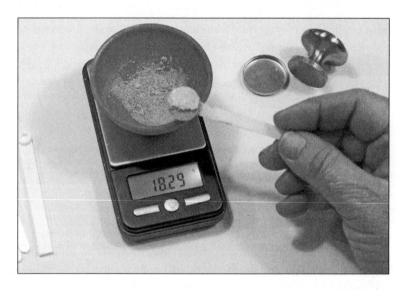

3. Grind the colorants for several seconds. Check your color by rubbing a little of the blend on the back of your hand. Make adjustments if needed.

4. Add the jojoba oil. Use a 3mm pipette to add 2 drops of preservative, and grind again. (For pressed shadow, use a 3mm pipette and add 6 extra drops jojoba oil.) Grind for 1 minute to ensure the liquids are well distributed throughout the dry colorants.

5. Fill your 10-milliliter sifter jar by spooning in a little shadow at a time. If you're pressing the powder, it's time to use the 6-inch dowel. Spoon half the shadow into the jar, press the dowel on top, and tap on the top of the dowel to press the shadow tight. Fill the jar with the rest of the shadow, and repeat tapping with the dowel. To have a full 10-gram jar of pressed eye shadow, you will need to double the recipe for the color grind.

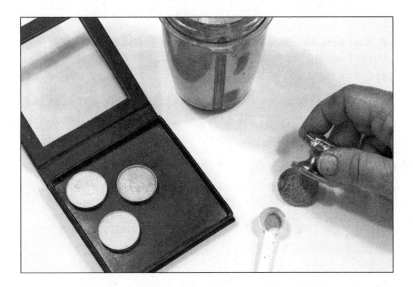

6. Place the lid on the jar, and store until you're ready to use. Or you can leave the eye shadow loose and use a spoon to fill the shifter jar.

IN THE MIRROR

The Egyptians believed that using dark colors on their eyelids not only enhanced their beauty but also warded off evil spirits.

Bright 'N' White Eye Shadow

A stark white shadow with a sparkle. Choose the Hilite mica that matches your eyes. This recipe makes enough grind to fill a 10-gram sifter jar.

Titanium dioxide	.1 ounce (2.8 grams)
Bismuth Oxychloride Diamond Sheen	.15 ounce (4.3 grams)
Hilite Green (for green eyes)	.15 ounce (4.3 grams)

Jojoba oil	⅛ teaspoon (.6 milliliter)
Preservative	2 drops

Prepare as directed in the Creamy White Eye Shadow recipe.

PRETTY POINTER

Personalize this recipe by using the Hilite that complements your eye color. For blue eyes, use Hilite Blue. For brown eyes, use Hilite Copper.

Peaches 'N' Cream Eye Shadow

A very light peach highlighter. This recipe makes enough grind to fill a 10-gram sifter jar.

Titanium dioxide	.2 ounce (5.7 grams)
Oriental Beige mica	.1 ounce (2.8 grams)
Butter Yellow mica	.2 ounce (5.7 grams)
Jojoba oil	⅛ teaspoon (.6 milliliter)
Preservative	2 drops

Prepare as directed in the Creamy White Eye Shadow recipe.

Highlighter for Dark Eyes

A light flesh tone highlighter with sparks to complement dark eye color. This recipe makes enough grind to fill a 10-gram sifter jar.

Titanium dioxide	.1 ounce (2.8 grams)
Ivory Lace mica	.15 ounce (4.3 grams)
Hilite Copper mica	.1 ounce (2.8 grams)
Jojoba oil	⅛ teaspoon (.6 milliliter)
Preservative	2 drops

Prepare as directed in the Creamy White Eye Shadow recipe.

Blues

Blue eye shadows make blue eyes look gorgeous. I've created a few gemstone blues that will be sure to please and will make your blue eyes seem even more intense.

Blue Gems Eye Shadow

A bright and intense gemstone blue. Use a brush to apply this shadow so you can control the intensity of the color. This recipe makes enough grind to fill a 10-gram sifter jar.

Blueberry Pop mica	.1 ounce (2.8 grams)
Sapphire mica	2 Tads
Blue Ferrocyanide	6 Tads
Jojoba oil	⅛ teaspoon (.6 milliliter)
Preservative	2 drops

Prepare as directed in the Creamy White Eye Shadow recipe.

Forget-Me-Not Eye Shadow

A beautiful and intense medium blue that has a flip of purple. This recipe makes enough grind to fill a 10-gram sifter jar.

Grape Pop mica	.1 ounce (2.8 grams)
Blueberry Pop mica	.1 ounce (2.8 grams)
Omega Blue mica	2 Dashes
Jojoba oil	⅛ teaspoon (.6 milliliter)
Preservative	2 drops

Prepare as directed in the Creamy White Eye Shadow recipe.

IN THE MIRROR

When a color has a flip, the color of the shadow changes slightly when you move and the light reflection changes. It flips to highlights of another color.

Blue Icicles Eye Shadow

A medium light blue with silver sparkle. This recipe makes enough grind to fill a 10-gram sifter jar.

Omega Blue oxide	2 Smidgens
Ferrocyanide oxide	2 Smidgens
Starlight Blue mica	.2 ounce (5.7 grams)
Jojoba oil	⅛ teaspoon (.6 milliliter)
Preservative	2 drops

Prepare as directed in the Creamy White Eye Shadow recipe.

Poppin' Blue Eye Shadow

A very intense blue with a satiny shine. When applying this shadow, use a brush, not a sponge applicator, so you don't overdo it—it's *that* intense. This recipe makes enough grind to fill a 10-gram sifter jar.

Grape Pop mica	.1 ounce (2.8 grams)
Colorona Dark Blue mica	.1 ounce (2.8 grams)
Omega Blue mica	1 Pinch
Jojoba oil	⅛ teaspoon (.6 milliliter)
Preservative	2 drops

Prepare as directed in the Creamy White Eye Shadow recipe.

Smokin' Steel Eye Shadow

A polished steel blue that's very intense. This shadow helps you blue-eyed folks create the smoky eye look. This recipe makes enough grind to fill a 10-gram sifter jar.

Blueberry Pop mica	.15 ounce (4.3 grams)
Steel Blue mica	.15 ounce (4.3 grams)
Jojoba oil	⅛ teaspoon (.6 milliliter)
Preservative	2 drops

Prepare as directed in the Creamy White Eye Shadow recipe.

Browns

Just about everyone can wear brown shadows. We give you several here to choose from.

Berry Brown Eye Shadow

A medium coppery brown with pink highlights. Not too dark for day wear, yet it works for evening, too. This recipe makes enough grind to fill a 10-gram sifter jar.

Dark Brown oxide	.02 ounce (.6 grams)
Artisan Coral mica	.25 ounce (7.1 grams)
Antique Copper mica	.07 ounce (2 grams)
Raspberry Pop mica	.32 ounce (9 grams)
Jojoba oil	⅛ teaspoon (.6 milliliter)
Preservative	2 drops

Prepare as directed in the Creamy White Eye Shadow recipe.

Smoky Brown Eye Shadow

A deep silvery brown. This is another shadow you can use to create the smoky eye look. This recipe makes enough grind to fill a 10-gram sifter jar.

Dark Brown oxide	.05 ounce (1.4 grams) plus 1 Dash
Black mica	.05 ounce (1.4 grams)
Grape Pop mica	.05 ounce (1.4 grams)
Bronze Fine mica	.2 ounce (5.7 grams)
Jojoba oil	⅛ teaspoon (.6 milliliter)
Preservative	2 drops

Prepare as directed in the Creamy White Eye Shadow recipe.

Deep Swiss Chocolate Eye Shadow

A deep and rich chocolate with fiery copper sparks. This will make beautiful smoky eyes. This recipe makes enough grind to fill a 10-gram sifter jar.

Dark Brown oxide	.1 ounce (2.8 grams)
Swiss Chocolate mica	.3 ounce (8.5 grams)

| Jojoba oil | ⅛ teaspoon (.6 milliliter) |
| Preservative | 2 drops |

Prepare as directed in the Creamy White Eye Shadow recipe.

Soft Brown Reflections Eye Shadow

A soft muted brown with a green flip. You look one way and it's a soft green, but look the other way and it's a soft brown. If you have hazel or green eyes, this shadow will look sensational on you! It's beautiful on brown eyes, too. This recipe makes enough grind to fill a 10-gram sifter jar.

Titanium dioxide	.1 ounce (2.8 grams)
Dragon Fly mica	.2 ounce (5.7 grams)
Jojoba oil	⅛ teaspoon (.6 milliliter)
Preservative	2 drops

Prepare as directed in the Creamy White Eye Shadow recipe.

Aladdin's Finery Eye Shadow

A medium tone but intense coppery brown with extra copper sparks. Perfect for day or evening wear. This recipe makes enough grind to fill a 10-gram sifter jar.

Aladdin's Lamp mica	.1 ounce (2.8 grams)
Bronze Fine mica	.1 ounce (2.8 grams)
TKB Trading Purely Matte Texture Base for Eyes	.1 ounce (2.8 grams)
Jojoba oil	⅛ teaspoon (.6 milliliter)
Preservative	2 drops

Prepare as directed in the Creamy White Eye Shadow recipe.

Greens

Green is one of my favorite colors. I've created several greens, from soft green to gemstone green. If you have green, hazel, or brown eyes, you'll surely find a goldmine of favorite shadows here!

Surrender to Me Eye Shadow

A medium sage green with a soft sheen that's perfect for day wear. This recipe makes enough grind to fill a 10-gram sifter jar.

Deep Green mica	.2 ounce (5.7 grams)
China Jade mica	.1 ounce (2.8 grams)
Gold Fine mica	.1 ounce (2.8 grams)
Jojoba oil	⅛ teaspoon (.6 milliliter)
Preservative	2 drops

Prepare as directed in the Creamy White Eye Shadow recipe.

Always and Forever Green Eye Shadow

A medium deep green with a satin sheen. If you have hazel eyes, this shadow will bring out all the green in your eyes. For green eyes, this shadow will make your green eyes very intense. This recipe makes enough grind to fill a 10-gram sifter jar.

Apple Green Pop mica	.1 ounce (2.8 grams)
Emerald mica	.2 ounce (5.7 grams)
TKB Trading Purely Matte Texture Base for Eyes	.1 ounce (2.8 grams)
Jojoba oil	⅛ teaspoon (.6 milliliter)
Preservative	2 drops

Prepare as directed in the Creamy White Eye Shadow recipe.

Softly Green Eye Shadow

A soft powdery green with a soft sparkle. It's a great green for daytime wear. This recipe makes enough grind to fill a 10-gram sifter jar.

Ocean Green mica	.2 ounce (5.7 grams)
Lotsa Lime mica	.1 ounce (2.8 grams)
TKB Trading Purely Matte Texture Base for Eyes	.1 ounce (2.8 grams)
Jojoba oil	⅛ teaspoon (.6 milliliter)
Preservative	2 drops

Prepare as directed in the Creamy White Eye Shadow recipe.

Ireland Eye Shadow

You'll be looking for the pot of gold with this eye shadow, a beautiful, intense green with a satin sheen. This recipe makes enough grind to fill a 10-gram sifter jar.

Apple Green Pop mica	.15 ounce (4.3 grams)
Lemon Drop Pop mica	.15 ounce (4.3 grams)
Emerald mica	.15 ounce (4.3 grams)
Jojoba oil	⅛ teaspoon (.6 milliliter)
Preservative	2 drops

Prepare as directed in the Creamy White Eye Shadow recipe.

Grays/Silvers

My daughter-in-law asked me to grind some gray shadows for her, so I did—and they look awesome! Both of these grinds have a lot of sparkle! Use them to help create that smoky eye look.

Silver Girl Eye Shadow

This is the lighter of the 2 silver gray shadows. It's less gray on the eyelid than what it looks in the jar—more of a silver than a gray. This recipe makes enough grind to fill a 10-gram sifter jar.

Polished Silver mica	.1 ounce (2.8 grams)
Black mica	.05 ounce (1.4 grams)
Black Amethyst mica	2 Dashes
TKB Trading Purely Matte Texture Base for Eyes	.1 ounce (2.8 grams)
Jojoba oil	⅛ teaspoon (.6 milliliter)
Preservative	2 drops

Prepare as directed in the Creamy White Eye Shadow recipe.

Smokin' Silver Eye Shadow

Smokin' Silver is a touch darker than Silver Girl, with a little more smoky gray. Use this color to contour the crease of the eyelid and to blend with Silver Girl on the outer edge of the eyelid to make the smoky eye look. This recipe makes enough grind to fill a 10-gram sifter jar.

Polished Silver	.1 ounce (2.8 grams)
Black mica	.1 ounce (2.8 grams)
Black Amethyst mica	.05 ounce (1.4 grams)
Jojoba oil	⅛ teaspoon (.6 milliliter)
Preservative	2 drops

Prepare as directed in the Creamy White Eye Shadow recipe.

Peaches

Peach shadows add a soft warmth to the eyes. I don't think there's any eye color that's not enhanced with a peach-colored eye shadow.

Rich and Deeply Peach Eye Shadow

A deep, dark, and intense peachy-brown tone. This shadow complements brown and hazel eyes beautifully. Rich and Deeply Peach is an intense shadow, so use a brush for application. This recipe makes enough grind to fill a 10-gram sifter jar.

Aladdin's Lamp mica	.2 ounce (5.7 grams)
Bronze Fine mica	.1 ounce (2.8 grams)
TKB Trading Purely Matte Texture Base for Eyes	.1 ounce (2.8 grams)
Jojoba oil	⅛ teaspoon (.6 milliliter)
Preservative	2 drops

Prepare as directed in the Creamy White Eye Shadow recipe.

Electric Peaches 'N' Oranges Eye Shadow

I think the name explains it very well. This grind has been approved by my teenage granddaughter. This recipe makes enough grind to fill a 10-gram sifter jar.

Tangerine Pop mica	.1 ounce (2.8 grams)
Umber mica	.1 ounce (2.8 grams)
Gold Fine mica	.025 ounce (.7 gram)
Sienna Fine mica	.05 ounce (1.4 grams)
Jojoba oil	⅛ teaspoon (.6 milliliter)
Preservative	2 drops

Prepare as directed in the Creamy White Eye Shadow recipe.

Soft Peach Eye Shadow

A soft and airy peach with a satin sheen. It's perfect for daytime and office wear. This recipe makes enough grind to fill a 10-gram sifter jar.

Artisan Coral mica	.2 ounce (5.7 grams)
Umber mica	.1 ounce (2.8 grams)
TKB Trading Purely Matte Texture Base for Eyes	.2 ounce (5.7 grams)
Jojoba oil	⅛ teaspoon (.6 milliliter)
Preservative	2 drops

Prepare as directed in the Creamy White Eye Shadow recipe.

Tibetan Peach Eye Shadow

A medium tone brown-peach with a satin sheen. This shadow makes hazel eyes pop and look sensational! This recipe makes enough grind to fill a 10-gram sifter jar.

Artisan Coral mica	.2 ounce (5.7 grams)
Tibetan Ochre mica	.1 ounce (2.8 grams)
TKB Trading Purely Matte Texture Base for Eyes	.1 ounce (2.8 grams)
Jojoba oil	⅛ teaspoon (.6 milliliter)
Preservative	2 drops

Prepare as directed in the Creamy White Eye Shadow recipe.

Purples

Purples and lavenders can make hazel, green, and brown eyes really pop. Even people with blue eyes can wear this color shadow. The darker purples are often used to create the smoky eye look.

Deep Purple Haze Eye Shadow

A strong and deep true purple. This shadow makes brown and green eyes pop! It's been granddaughter approved. This recipe makes enough grind to fill a 10-gram sifter jar.

Black oxide	.15 ounce (4.3 grams)
Ultramarine Violet mica	.05 ounce (1.4 grams)
Black mica	.05 ounce (1.4 grams)
Grape Pop mica	.25 ounce (7.1 grams)
Jojoba oil	⅛ teaspoon (.6 milliliter)
Preservative	2 drops

Prepare as directed in the Creamy White Eye Shadow recipe.

Deep and Smoky Purple Eye Shadow

An intense smoky and deep purple. This shadow is the one you must have to create hypnotic, smoky eyes. It's granddaughter approved, and the one she asks for the most. This recipe makes enough grind to fill a 10-gram sifter jar.

Dark Brown oxide	2 Dashes
Black Amethyst mica	.2 ounce (5.7 grams)
Grape Pop mica	.2 ounce (5.7 grams)
Black mica	2 Dashes
Jojoba oil	⅛ teaspoon (.6 milliliter)
Preservative	2 drops

Prepare as directed in the Creamy White Eye Shadow recipe.

Purple Fog Eye Shadow

A pewter purple with a satin sheen. It's light and has more of a pewter tone than purple. This recipe makes enough grind to fill a 10-gram sifter jar.

Titanium dioxide	.05 ounce (1.4 grams)
Patagonia Purple mica	.2 ounce (5.7 grams)

Pearl White mica	.05 ounce (1.4 grams)
Jojoba oil	⅛ teaspoon (.6 milliliter)
Preservative	2 drops

Prepare as directed in the Creamy White Eye Shadow recipe.

Purple People Eater Eye Shadow

A soft and airy purple. This shadow is great for daytime wear, even to the office. And it's soft enough for young teen girls who are just starting to wear a little makeup. This recipe makes enough grind to fill a 10-gram sifter jar.

Titanium dioxide	.05 ounce (1.4 grams)
Grape Pop mica	.15 ounce (4.3 grams)
Pearl White mica	.15 ounce (4.3 grams)
Jojoba oil	⅛ teaspoon (.6 milliliter)
Preservative	2 drops

Prepare as directed in the Creamy White Eye Shadow recipe.

Teals

I could play with these eye shadows all day long and not get tired of this color group. They are perfect for those with blue or green eyes.

Teal Me Eye Shadow

A very bright and intense teal with a lot of sparkle. The Turquoise Tweak mica adds all the sparkle. Use a brush to apply this intense shadow. This recipe makes enough grind to fill a 10-gram sifter jar.

Turquoise Tweak mica	.1 ounce (2.8 grams)
Coral Reef Blue mica	.1 ounce (2.8 grams)
Blueberry Pop mica	.1 ounce (2.8 grams)
Apple Green Pop mica	.1 ounce (2.8 grams)
Jojoba oil	⅛ teaspoon (.6 milliliter)
Preservative	2 drops

Prepare as directed in the Creamy White Eye Shadow recipe.

Teal We Meet Again Eye Shadow

A medium and soft teal tone with a sparkle. This recipe makes enough grind to fill a 10-gram sifter jar.

Totally Teal mica	.2 ounce (5.7 grams)
Sparkle mica	.1 ounce (2.8 grams)
Turquoise Tweak mica	1 Tad
Jojoba oil	⅛ teaspoon (.6 milliliter)
Preservative	2 drops

Prepare as directed in the Creamy White Eye Shadow recipe.

Deep Teal Waters Eye Shadow

A deep teal with more green than blue with a satin sheen. This is another shadow you'll want to use a brush to apply. This recipe makes enough grind to fill a 10-gram sifter jar.

Blue Steel mica	.15 ounce (4.3 grams)
Coral Reef Blue mica	.05 ounce (1.4 grams)
Pennsylvania Green mica	.05 ounce (1.4 grams)
Blueberry Pop mica	.05 ounce (1.4 grams)
Jojoba oil	⅛ teaspoon (.6 milliliter)
Preservative	2 drops

Prepare as directed in the Creamy White Eye Shadow recipe.

Sparkling Turquoise Eye Shadow

The name says it all—bright and sparking! This recipe makes enough grind to fill a 10-gram sifter jar.

Blueberry Pop mica	.15 ounce (4.3 grams)
Apple Green Pop mica	.1 ounce (2.8 grams)
Turquoise Tweak mica	.05 ounce (1.4 grams)
Jojoba oil	⅛ teaspoon (.6 milliliter)
Preservative	2 drops

Prepare as directed in the Creamy White Eye Shadow recipe.

Making Eyeliner

Eyeliner isn't hard to make. But when your family and friends see the liners you've made, they'll be very surprised and amazed that you got the liner in that tiny hole. (I won't tell them how easy it is if you won't.)

You can make several kinds of eyeliner:

- Pressed
- Pencils
- Liquid

In this section, I teach you how to make each type.

Many of the eye shadow color grinds make wonderful pencil eyeliners. For a smoky look, try using the Deep and Smokey Purple or Purple Haze color grind. If you want something green, use Always and Forever Green. Play with the grinds until you find one you love for eyeliner.

Here's what you need to make eyeliner:

- Stove or microwave
- Scale
- Coffee grinder or mortar and pestle
- Small saucepan or heat-resistant glass container
- Stainless-steel measuring spoons
- Several small glass or plastic bowls
- Syringe, with no needle
- 2 spoons
- 3mm pipettes
- Latex gloves
- Face mask

- Waxed paper

- 10-gram sifter jar

- 6-inch dowel rod

- Fillable eyeliner pencils that can be sharpened (These have a hole down the center and look like a pencil.)

- Fillable eyeliner tubes with brush wand

PRETTY POINTER

Check out makingcosmetics.com for the fillable eyeliner pencils. TKB Trading has the eyeliner and mascara tubes, as well as the sifter jars, in all sizes. (See Appendix D.)

Eyeliner Pencil

You have to work quickly while filling the pencils. The mixture cools fast, and it has to be hot enough for you to push it all the way to the bottom of the pencil. Don't worry about the spills or leaks; both are to be expected. Store any leftovers in a zipper-lock bag for later use. This recipe makes 1 ounce (28.4 grams), or enough to fill 8 eyeliner pencils.

Beeswax	.1 ounce (2.8 grams)
Candelilla wax	.2 ounce (5.7 grams)
Palm kernel stearin	.2 ounce (5.7 grams)
Jojoba oil	.2 ounce (5.7 grams)
Castor oil	.2 ounce (5.7 grams)
Color grind	.1 ounce (2.8 grams)
Preservative	.01 ounce (0.3 gram)

1. Place a small bowl or cup on the scale and push the tare button to zero out the weight of the container. Weigh the waxes and the oils, transferring each to a small saucepan or a microwave-safe bowl. Heat over low heat or in the microwave for short cook times on medium power until the mixture is melted.

2. When all the wax has melted, remove from heat. Add the color grind, and stir well. Add the preservative, and stir well again.

3. Put a piece of clean paper or waxed paper on the counter in front of you. Using the syringe, draw up at least 3 milliliters mixture. Hold the eyeliner pencil upright with one end flat on the paper. Put the tip of the syringe against the hole in the top of the pencil, and push the plunger until the mixture starts coming back out. Prop the pencil upright in a cup to dry. Repeat with remaining pencils.

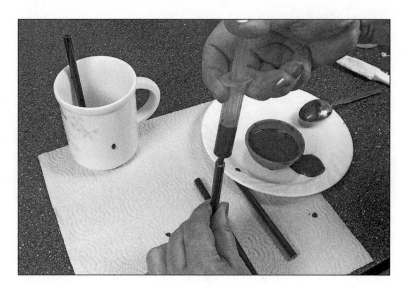

4. Let pencils set until the next day. Sharpen, and they're ready to use!

PRETTY POINTER

You can divide the mixture in half so you can use two different color grinds. But I don't recommend making a batch of eyeliner smaller than 1 ounce (28.4 grams) for the pencils. There's not enough mixture at that amount to remain hot long enough to fill more than 1 pencil before you'll have to melt the mixture again. And at that point, there just isn't enough left to work with. You can fill 8 pencils from 1 ounce eyeliner base.

Pressed Powder Eyeliner

To have a full 10-gram sifter jar of eyeliner, you need to double the color grind recipe. There may be a smidge left over, but at least the jar will be full. When following the recipe for a color grind, do not add the jojoba oil and preservative. You will add a different amount of those ingredients for making the pressed eyeliner rather than eye shadow. Just follow this recipe. This recipe makes .36 ounce (10.2 grams) and enough to fill a 10-gram sifter jar.

Oxide or color grind (your choice)	.7 ounce (19.8 grams)
Jojoba oil	⅛ teaspoon (.6 milliliter) plus 6 drops
Preservative	4 drops

1. Follow the instructions for weighing the micas and oxides to make a color grind, or just use black oxide.

2. With your coffee grinder or in your mortar and pestle, grind the oxide or color grind. Then add the increased amount of jojoba oil and preservative. Be sure everything is well incorporated.

3. Fill your jar with half the mixture. Press with the dowel until the mixture is firm. Fill the jar with the remaining mixture, and repeat tapping with the dowel.

IN THE MIRROR

The ancient Egyptian women first started making eyeliner from burnt almonds, soot, lead, and copper. Both women and men used the makeup.

Liquid Eyeliner

This recipe isn't as hard to make as it looks. Just roll up your sleeves and give it a try. You can use any of the oxides or micas, including the color grinds, to make eyeliner. Have fun and create a few wild sparkly liners with the micas for holidays or Halloween. This recipe makes 1 ounce (28.4 grams), or enough to fill 2 eyeliner tubes.

The colorant:

Oxide or color grind	1 teaspoon (4.9 milliliters)
Magnesium stearate	1 teaspoon (4.9 milliliters)
Sericite mica	1 teaspoon (4.9 milliliters)

The waxes and oil:

Candelilla wax	½ teaspoon (2.5 milliliters)
Beeswax	½ teaspoon (2.5 milliliters)
Stearic acid	½ teaspoon (2.5 milliliters)
Jojoba oil	1½ tablespoons (22.5 milliliters)
Preservative	(see manufacturer's recommendation)

1. Start by measuring your oxide or color grind, magnesium stearate, and sericite mica. Place them in a small bowl, and set aside.

2. Measure your waxes and jojoba oil, and put them in a small saucepan or a heat-resistant glass container. If using a stove, set pan over the lowest heat and slowly melt the waxes. If using a microwave, use short heating times set at half power.

3. When the waxes have completely melted, add the colorant mixture. Stir well and use a syringe to fill the eyeliner tubes.

4. Allow to cure for 5 to 7 days before use. Apply to powdered eyelids.

SAFETY FIRST

You'll notice that this recipe is in a different format from other recipes. That's because it works only when you carefully measure the ingredients. This is a very advanced recipe, and you should wait to tackle it only after you've made many of the other recipes in this book. Rely on your knowledge of cooking to help you navigate through the instructions and technique of making this liquid eyeliner and the following mascara.

Making Mascara

The mascaras on the market today are made with chemicals and preservatives that contain formaldehyde or parabens. We pay a high price for these waterproof, lash-lengthening formulas. Although the following mascara recipe isn't waterproof and won't add length to your lashes, it is natural and free of any harmful chemicals.

When making mascara, you must work quickly before the gel gets too thick, which makes it hard to fill the tube. It took me several tries to get one filled. Oh, and it can be very messy. Be sure to cover your work surface with waxed paper.

You make this recipe in several parts. Read the entire recipe carefully before you start. While you're melting the waxes, you'll also be working on the water phase.

Here's what you need to make mascara:

- 2 small saucepans

- Stove with 2 burners

- Scale

- Syringe, with no needle (Look for one with a big hole in the end for drawing up this thickish gel.)

- Several mascara tubes
- A couple spoons or a tiny whisk
- Small cups or bowls
- Fillable mascara tubes
- Paper towels—lots

PRETTY POINTER

If your mascara dries out before you've had a chance to use it up, add a few drops of olive oil and twist the wand around to help loosen the mascara inside the tube. Let the olive oil soak into the mascara and then you'll be able to continue using it.

Mascara

Do not try to make more than this 2-ounce recipe at a time. The mascara will become too thick before you can fill all the tubes. You will use an oil of your choice to "wet" the oxide so it can be added to your formulation without any lumps or clumps. This oil can be any of your favorite oils, even glycerin if you prefer. This recipe makes 2 ounces (56.7 grams), or enough to fill 3 or 4 mascara tubes.

The color:

Oxide or color grind	.1 ounce (2.8 grams)
Wetting oil (your choice)	.05 ounce (1.4 grams)

IN THE MIRROR

Just like in cooking, you have to wet a dry ingredient to add it to a liquid. You have to do that in this recipe with the oxide so it dissolves quicker when it's added to the melted waxes. I like to use sweet almond oil.

The waxes:

Candelilla wax	.15 ounce (4.3 grams)
Beeswax	.1 ounce (2.8 grams)
Emulsifying or polar wax	.1 ounce (2.8 grams)
Stearic acid	.1 ounce (2.8 grams)

The water and thickeners:

Distilled water	1.4 ounces (39.7 grams)
Aloe vera gel (or your choice)	.06 ounce (1.7 grams)
Jojoba oil	.05 ounce (1.4 grams)
Glycerin	.05 ounce (1.4 grams)
HEC	.03 ounce (.9 gram)

Just before you fill the tubes, add:

Preservative	.02 ounce (.6 gram)

1. Put a small cup or bowl on your scale and push the tare button to zero out the weight of the container. Weigh your oxide or color grind. Remove the container from the scale. Weigh the wetting oil in another bowl, and add to the colorant. Stir well, ensuring the oil is well distributed throughout the colorant. Set aside.

2. Weigh the waxes, and put them in the first saucepan. Set them aside for now.

3. Now put another small container or cup on the scale and again push the tare button. Weigh the water, aloe vera or other oil, jojoba oil, and glycerin. Add those to the second saucepan.

4. Now put another small container or cup on the scale, push the tare button, and weigh the HEC. Set the HEC aside for now.

5. Set both saucepans over the lowest heat. Slowly melt the waxes while you heat the water. When the water mixture is warm and the waxes in the other pan are almost melted, remove the water pan from the heat and add the HEC. Stir until it's completely dissolved.

6. Add the oxide mixture to the melted waxes, and stir well. Remember to work quickly!

BEAUTY BIT

HEC (Hydroxyethylcellulose) is a water-soluble thickener used in cosmetics. It's a natural substance that comes from cellulose (paper).

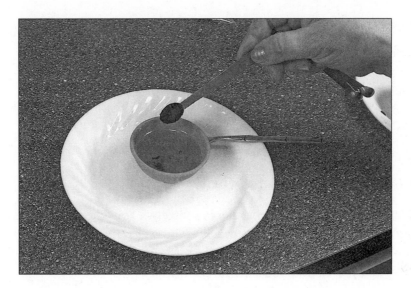

7. Add the water mixture to the wax mixture, and stir. It will get all lumpy. Return the saucepan to the stove and over medium-low, stir until it all comes together. It may take a few minutes to get the mixture hot enough to come together, but be patient and give it time to do its thing. Don't rush it. Remove from heat and continue stirring. Now add the preservative, and mix well again.

8. Fill the mascara tubes using a syringe. Tap them on the counter to be sure no air is caught in the tubes as you fill them. Leave a little space at the top so you can insert the brush and screw it down into the tube.

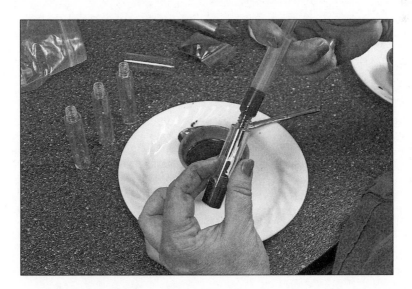

9. Let the mascara cure for 4 or 5 days before use.

Enjoy your new natural mascara!

For good eyelash conditioner, mix equal parts of two or three oils such as grapeseed, apricot kernel, and sweet almond oils, and apply a light coating to eyelashes at night before bed. You can also condition your eyelashes using castor oil jelly.

The Least You Need to Know

- It's easy and so much fun to make eye shadows. Your choices of colors are nearly limitless!
- When working with micas and oxides, especially in such tiny amounts as are necessary for eye shadows, you'll need a good scale.
- Oxides and micas are messy! Wear old clothes when working with them, and be sure to cover your work surface with waxed paper to help with cleanup.

Everything Lips

In This Chapter

- Create the perfect lipstick shade, whatever the occasion
- DIY lipsticks with matching lip liner pencils
- Making moisturizing lip balms

I love making lip products! They're so easy and inexpensive to make. In this chapter, we give you several recipes to try—and enjoy!

Making Lip Balms

When making lip balm, the most important thing to remember is the butters you use can become grainy if they're melted too quickly and get too hot. The best way to melt the butter is over *low* heat. Don't let the butter completely melt while on the burner. Instead, remove the butter from the heat when a few unmelted pieces still remain. Stir the butter until the rest of the pieces melt.

In these recipes, you can always change any of the butters for one of your choosing. That's also true for the oils. However, please swap a butter for a butter and an oil for an oil. That way the firmness of the balm remains consistent.

Now what about flavor? While shopping for lip product ingredients, you might find lip balm flavor oils. These oils don't actually have a taste, but they do have a scent, which tricks your brain into thinking the lip balm tastes like it smells. Even though they say "lip balm flavor," they can also be added to your lipsticks. How about making a bright red lipstick using apple lip balm flavoring?

You can use honey to flavor your lip balm, but I advise you to use honey powder and not actual honey. Honey tends to become grainy in lip balms, while the powder doesn't.

Be careful not to get the cocoa butter too hot because it also tends to become grainy, and after a month or two, little crystallized buds of cocoa butter pop up on the top of the lip balm. Instead, melt the cocoa butter over low heat slowly. Remove it from heat before it has finished melting, and continue stirring until the butter has completely melted.

For an extra-special touch, you can add a small amount of one of the sparkly micas to your lip balm. It won't color your lips, but it will add a nice visual touch.

I recommend that you use Optiphen Plus as your preservative. It's paraben- and formaldehyde-free. The use rate is 1 percent.

SAFETY FIRST

Always clean your workspace before you begin. Wipe the counter with alcohol or 3 percent hydrogen peroxide. Sterilize all your equipment, including your containers. It's helpful to keep a bottle of alcohol handy while you work for wiping down utensils as you may need them.

Here's what you need to make lip balm:

- Lip balm tubes
- Latex gloves
- Alcohol or hydrogen peroxide
- Scale
- Set of 5 TKB Trading stainless-steel measuring spoons (Tad, Dash, Pinch, Smidgen, and Drop sizes)
- Regular measuring spoons
- Spoons
- Small cup or bowl
- Stove or microwave
- Small saucepan or a microwavable glass measuring cup
- Syringe, without needle, or 1-cup (236.6-milliliter) measuring cup

Before you begin, be sure to sterilize your lip balm tubes with a commercial sanitizing product or alcohol and let them completely air-dry. Store in a baggie if you are going to wait a few days before using them. Otherwise, have them lined up in a row before you begin.

Shea-Ya-Like Lip Balm

With the shea butter and sweet almond oil, this balm will keep your lips soft and moist all year round. It's a basic lip balm recipe that works for all types of lip needs. This recipe makes 4 ounces (113.4 grams) lip balm, or enough to fill 25 (.15-ounce; 4.3-gram) lip balm tubes.

White beeswax	1 ounce (28.4 grams)
Soy wax (We use Joy Wax.)	1.5 ounces (42.5 grams)
Cosmetic-grade shea butter	.5 ounce (14.2 grams)
Sweet almond oil	.5 ounce (14.2 grams)
Jojoba oil	.5 ounce (14.2 grams)
Flavor oil	1 teaspoon (4.9 milliliters; or to taste)
Preservative	.04 ounce (1.1 grams)

1. Place a small bowl on your scale, and push the tare button to zero out the weight of the bowl. Weigh each of your waxes and butter, and place them in the saucepan or microwave-safe container.

2. Melt the waxes and butter over low heat. If heating in the microwave, use half power for 1 minute at a time. Be careful not to overheat your butters.

3. While the waxes and butter melt, weigh the oils and add them to the melting wax mixture. When the waxes and butter are almost totally melted, remove from heat and stir while they finish melting.

4. Now add the lip balm flavoring and preservative. Stir until everything is well incorporated.

5. Using a syringe or a glass measuring cup, carefully fill the lip balm tubes to the very top. Let cool until hard (the cooler the room, the quicker they harden) before you place caps on top.

Bee Sweet Lip Balm

With the addition of grapeseed oil, this lip balm recipe has more conditioning than the Shea-Ya–Like recipe. This is a good winter balm to prevent chapped lips. If you want, you can omit the soy wax and increase the beeswax to 5 ounces (141.7 grams). This recipe can be cut in half down to 2 ounces (56.7 grams) or doubled to make any size batch you want. This recipe makes 8 ounces (226.8 grams) lip balm, or enough to fill 50 (.15-ounce; 4.3-gram) lip balm tubes.

White beeswax	3 ounces (85 grams)
Soy wax	2 ounces (56.7 grams)
Cosmetic-grade shea butter	1 ounce (28.4 grams)
Grapeseed oil	.5 ounce (14.2 grams)
Sweet almond oil	.5 ounce (14.2 grams)
Jojoba oil	1 ounce (28.4 grams)
Flavor oil	1 teaspoon (4.9 milliliters; or to taste)
Preservative	.08 ounce (2.3 grams)

Prepare as directed in the Shea-Ya–Like Lip Balm recipe.

IN THE MIRROR

Mowrah butter is my all-time favorite butter to use in lip balms and lipsticks, but it has become impossible to find. Several years of bad crops have led to a shortage of this wonderfully healing and soothing butter. Hopefully we will see this butter on the market again in the future. When and if that happens, do yourself a favor and buy some of the ultra-refined mowrah butter and add it to your lip balm recipe.

Cocoa Buttery Lip Balm

This lip balm is my favorite. It has all the oils mature skin needs plus the butters to heal and protect your lips. You can cut this recipe down to as little as 2 ounces or increase it to whatever size batch you want to make. Take special care when melting the cocoa butter. If you're unable to get Joy Wax, use white beeswax instead. This recipe makes 8 ounces (226.8 grams), or enough to fill 50 (.15-ounce; 4.3-gram) lip balm tubes.

Candelilla wax	2 ounces (56.7 grams)
Joy Wax (soy wax blend)	3 ounces (85 grams)
Cocoa butter	.5 ounce (14.2 grams)
Cosmetic-grade shea butter	1 ounce (28.4 grams)
Sweet almond oil	.5 ounce (14.2 grams)
Pumpkin seed oil	.5 ounce (14.2 grams)
Evening primrose oil	.5 ounce (14.2 grams)
Preservative	.08 ounce (2.3 grams)

Prepare as directed in the Shea-Ya–Like Lip Balm recipe.

Making Lip Gloss

I don't know any girl—young or not-so-young!—who doesn't love lip gloss. And as a bonus: it's one of the easiest cosmetics to make! You can make a really simple gloss using glycerin and castor oil, or you can add more ingredients, creating a gloss that conditions while adding shine and maybe a touch of color. Lip-safe micas are a simple way to add color. How much you add determines how much color sticks to your lips.

Many commercial-flavor oils are available for use in lip products. You can mix these together or use them as they are. I often mix chocolate and mint flavor oils for lip balm and gloss. These flavor oils don't actually have a taste, only the scent, which tricks your nose into "tasting" the flavor.

Package your finished gloss in roll-on bottles or bottles with a fuzzy-tipped wand.

Here's what you need to make lip gloss:

- ⅓-ounce (9.4-gram) roll-on bottles (sterilized)
- Small microwave-safe bowl, small saucepan, or glass measuring cup
- Scale
- Tiny funnel
- Microwave or stove
- Spoon

Simple and Conditioning Lip Gloss

This very simple recipe is a snap to make, and it offers wonderful conditioning for your lips and keeps them kissably soft. This recipe makes 2 ounces (56.7 grams), or enough to fill 6 (⅓-ounce; 9.4-gram) lip gloss bottles.

Castor oil	.3 ounce (8.5 grams)
Sweet almond oil	.5 ounce (14.2 grams)
Jojoba oil (clear)	.2 ounce (5.7 grams)
Candelilla wax (or your choice)	.3 ounce (8.5 grams)
Glycerin	.5 ounce (14.2 grams)
Vitamin E	.2 ounce (5.7 grams)
Preservative	(see manufacturer's recommendation)
Flavor oil	¼ teaspoon (1.2 milliliters; or to taste)
Lip-safe mica (optional)	.1 ounce (2.8 grams)

1. Place a bowl on your scale, and push the tare button. Weigh your oils and wax one at a time. Place in a microwave-safe bowl or in a small saucepan.

2. If using a microwave oven, heat on half power, in short spurts (about 30 seconds), until all the wax has melted. If using the stovetop, melt over low heat until all the wax has melted. Remove from heat.

3. Let mixture cool slightly before adding the preservative, flavoring, and color. Stir well.

4. Using a tiny funnel, fill the lip gloss bottles. Let completely cool before screwing on the roller and lids.

Colorful Lip Gloss

Lip gloss only leaves a hint of color on your lips, but sometimes a hint is all you need or want. If you'd like a little more color, increase the mica to .2 ounces (5.7 grams). This recipe makes 2 ounces (56.7 grams), or enough to fill 6 (⅓-ounce; 9.4-gram) lip gloss bottles.

Oil (your choice)	.5 ounce (14.2 grams)
Castor oil	.3 ounce (8.5 grams)
Jojoba oil	.2 ounce (5.7 grams)
Cocoa butter	.3 ounce (8.5 grams)
Candelilla wax (or your choice)	.4 ounce (11.3 grams)
Vitamin E	.2 ounce (5.7 grams)
Preservative	(see manufacturer's recommendation)
Flavor oil	¼ teaspoon (1.2 grams; or to taste)
Lip-safe mica	.1 ounce (2.8 grams)

Prepare as directed in the Simple and Conditioning Lip Gloss recipe.

Lava Lip Gloss

This is not our recipe, but one many hand-crafters use for making this fun lip gloss. The gloss will separate, and the colored glycerin will settle at the bottom of the bottle—just like the lava lamps from the 1960s! Turn the bottle over several times to mix color and clear together. This recipe makes 3 ounces (85 grams), or enough to fill 9 (⅓-ounce; 9.4-gram) lip gloss bottles.

Glycerin	1.4 ounces (39.7 grams)
Lip-safe mica	.05 ounce (1.4 grams)

Castor oil	1.4 ounces (39.7 grams)
Vitamin E	.15 ounce (4.3 grams)
Preservative	(see manufacturer's recommendation)
Flavor oil	½ teaspoon (2.4 grams; or to taste)

1. Place a bowl on the scale, and push the tare button. Weigh the glycerin and mica. In a small bowl or measuring cup, pour the glycerin over the mica, and stir until the mica has dissolved in the glycerin.

2. Place another bowl on the scale, and push the tare button. Weigh the castor oil and vitamin E, and add them to the glycerin mixture. Stir well.

3. Put the bowl back on the scale, and push the tare button again. Weigh the preservative, and add it to the glycerin. Add the flavor oil, and stir well.

4. Using the tiny funnel, pour the gloss into the bottles. Cap and have fun!

Making Lipsticks

I could stay locked in my workshop for a month just playing with blends for lipstick. My mother once said the older the woman, the redder her lipstick. Well, that's not exactly true these days, or in the last 20 or so years. During my 20s and 30s, I wore very red lipstick and loved it. Nowadays, I wear very light shades, so I guess the trends have reversed. No matter what your color choice, we give you several color grinds we hope you'll love.

If you don't find your perfect shade among the recipes in this section, we also show you how to grind your own personal favorite.

PRETTY POINTER

You can use lip balm tubes for your lipstick and pour the mixture directly into the tube. After the lipstick hardens, just cut the end at a slant. If you want to use lipstick tubes, you'll need a mold. Several types are available. TKB Trading carries the professional metal 12-stick molds, which are very expensive, or you can buy a plastic single- or triple-stick mold from Making Cosmetics. Both companies have online stores.

You'll need to keep in mind a few pointers before you start. You need to have either lanolin or castor oil jelly in your recipe for the color to stick to your lips. You also need to have a tiny amount of oxide in all the grinds. If you omit these, your lipstick won't color your lips. I don't like the smell or taste of the castor oil jelly, so I use lanolin in the recipes. Some people use Vaseline in place of the lanolin. Or I have a recipe for making a natural jelly instead.

If you don't add enough color grind to the lipstick, it won't coat your lips. If the lipstick is too hard—guess what—it won't leave color on your lips. If you have too much color grind, the lipstick will be brittle and cakey and even contain cracks. Your lipstick needs curing time, at least a few weeks.

It's important to follow the recipes carefully. Once you're comfortable with what you're doing, you can tweak the recipes and make them your own.

Here's what you need to make lipsticks:

- Small saucepan or microwaveable container
- Scale
- Stove or microwave
- Spoons
- 3mm pipettes
- Small paper cups
- Set of 5 TKB Trading stainless-steel measuring spoons (Tad, Dash, Pinch, Smidgen, and Drop sizes)
- Lipstick tubes and a lipstick mold, or lip balm tubes (You can pour the lipstick directly into the lip balm tubes.)

Be sure your area is clean and your lipstick tubes or lip balm tubes have been sterilized and are in a baggie ready for use.

Lip-Loving Lipstick

This is my favorite lipstick because it glides on so smoothly. In the recipe, I use Joy Wax instead of beeswax. This is a personal choice, and if you'd rather use beeswax, it works well, too. This recipe makes 2 ounces (56.7 grams), or 12 lipsticks in (.15-ounce; 4.3-gram) lip balm tubes.

Joy Wax, soy wax, or beeswax	.2 ounce (5.7 grams)
Candelilla wax	.3 ounce (8.5 grams)
Evening primrose oil	.2 ounce (5.7 grams)
Macadamia oil	.2 ounce (5.7 grams)
Castor oil	.5 ounce (14.2 grams)
Lanolin (or castor oil jelly or Vaseline)	.2 ounce (5.7 grams)
Vitamin E	.1 ounce (2.8 grams)

Cosmetic-grade shea butter	.2 ounce (5.7 grams)
Color grind	.2 to .4 ounce (5.7 to 11.3 grams)
Preservative	.02 ounce (.6 grams)

1. Set your scale to ounces or grams. Place your small cup or bowl on the scale, and push the tare button to zero out the weight of the container. Weigh each of the waxes, pushing the tare button each time to zero out the weight of the container. Transfer each wax to a small saucepan or microwavable container. Melt them over low heat or in the microwave on half power in 1-minute intervals.

2. Weigh your oils, lanolin, vitamin E, and butter. Add them to the waxes, and slowly melt the butter. Just before all the butter has melted, remove from heat and stir until the butter has completely melted. This prevents the butter from becoming grainy in the lipstick after it has hardened.

3. Weigh your color grind and preservative, and add them to the mixture. Stir until all the color is incorporated.

4. Pour mixture into mold or tubes. Remelt if necessary until all your tubes or molds are full.

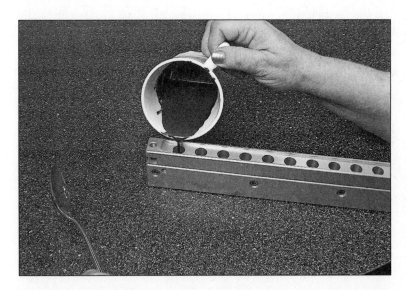

5. Let the lipstick harden in the refrigerator for 2 hours. If you used lip balm tubes, cut the top of the lipstick at a slant.

Here's how to load lipstick tubes from a lipstick mold:

1. Separate the lipstick mold.

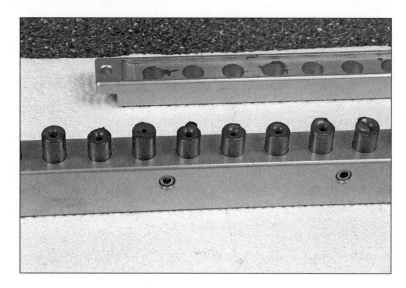

2. With the lipstick tube rolled all the way up, place it over the bottom end of the lipstick, and gently press the tube down over the lipstick. You may want to gently loosen the lipstick before you slide the tube over it.

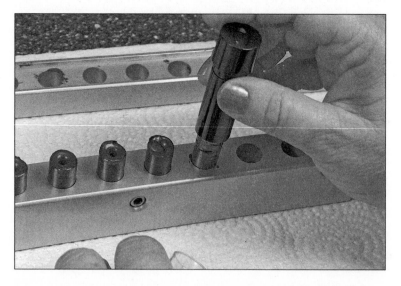

3. Gently pull up. The lipstick will pull away from the mold and load perfectly into the tube. Roll down the tube, and place the cap on. Easy!

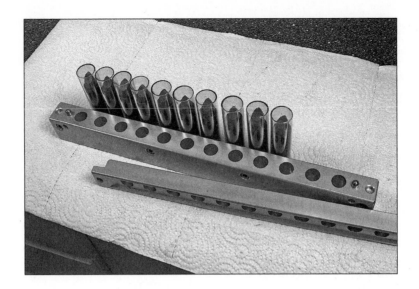

Mango Lipstick

Thanks to the conditioning of mango butter and pumpkin seed oil, this lipstick keeps your lips moist and soft. This recipe makes a little harder lipstick. Depending on where you live, the harder the lipstick, the less likely it is to melt. We live in Texas, and everyone knows how hot it can get during the summer months. We have to be careful not to make it too hard. That causes a whole set of other problems! This recipe makes 2 ounces (56.7 grams), or 12 (.15-ounce; 4.3-gram) lipsticks.

White beeswax	.3 ounce (8.5 grams)
Candelilla wax	.2 ounce (5.7 grams)
Palm kernel stearin	.2 ounce (5.7 grams)
Pumpkin seed oil	.2 ounce (5.7 grams)
Jojoba oil	.2 ounce (5.7 grams)
Castor oil	.5 ounce (14.2 grams)
Lanolin (or castor oil jelly or Vaseline)	.1 ounce (2.8 grams)
Mango butter	.1 ounce (2.8 grams)
Color grind	.2 ounce (5.7 grams)
Preservative	.02 ounce (.6 gram)

Prepare as directed in the Lip-Loving Lipstick recipe.

BEAUTY BIT

Palm kernel stearin is a solid natural fat, a by-product from refining palm olein. In lipstick, it adds hardness while also helping the color glide onto the lips.

Making Color Grinds for Lipsticks

We've created some wonderful color grinds for you to use in your lipsticks. Some of these grinds work well for blushes as well—maybe you remember seeing a few of them in that chapter. You can also match your lipstick and lip liner pencil using the same color grind in both. Each of these grinds makes just enough colorant for one lipstick recipe.

Here's what you need to make color grinds for lipsticks:

- Scale
- Stove or microwave oven
- Small saucepan or microwavable bowl
- Alcohol or hydrogen peroxide
- Paper towels
- Small paper cups
- Spoons
- 3mm pipettes
- Facemask
- Latex gloves
- Waxed paper
- Coffee grinder or mortar and pestle

> **IN THE MIRROR**
>
> Where you see the words *Tad, Dash, Pinch, Smidgen,* and *Drop,* know these refer to the set of 5 stainless-steel measuring spoons sold at TKB Trading. I use these for the really tiny amounts of color.

Browns and Cinnamons

This is one of my favorite groups! I had to limit myself to these recipes; otherwise, this chapter would have been full of brown and cinnamon recipes! Everyone can wear browns and cinnamons. They look fantastic for daytime or nighttime wear.

My 'd Azure Lipstick Color Grind

A chocolate brown with red and pink highlights. This recipe makes your lips look delicious and sexy. It can be worn day or night for that perfect touch. You may want to double it if you want stronger color in your lipstick. This recipe makes .2 ounce (5.7 grams) color grind.

Cote'd Azure mica	.1 ounce (2.8 grams)
Swiss Chocolate mica	.05 ounce (1.4 grams)
Crucible Red mica	.05 ounce (1.4 grams)
Red #170 or red oxide	1 Drop

1. Place a piece of waxed paper on the counter in front of you.

2. Set your scale to grams or ounces. Place your small cup or bowl on the scale, and push the tare button. This will zero out the weight of the container.

3. Weigh the first oxide or mica. Transfer it to your coffee grinder or mortar and pestle. Put the cup or bowl back on the scale, and again push the tare button. Continue weighing each colorant until you have each one transferred into the grinder and ready to grind.

4. Grind the colorant together for several seconds. Check your color by rubbing a little of the blend on the back of your hand.

5. If you're not planning on using the color grind right away, store it in a zipper-lock bag until ready to use.

Sensuous Lipstick Color Grind

A deep brownish-red with a satin sheen—seriously red, hot, and a must-have for winter or evening wear. This recipe makes .25 ounce (7.1 grams) color grind.

Red oxide—blue shade	.1 ounce (2.8 grams)
Antique Copper mica	.1 ounce (2.8 grams)
Autumn Leaves Sparks mica	.05 ounce (1.4 grams)

Prepare as directed in the My 'd Azure Lipstick Color Grind recipe.

Cinnamon Fire Lipstick Color Grind

A cinnamon red with copper sparks. This is one of my favorite lip colors for when I go out; it goes with just about anything. This recipe makes .25 ounce (7.1 grams) color grind.

Queen Kathryn mica	.1 ounce (2.8 grams)
Antique Copper mica	.1 ounce (2.8 grams)
Burning Leaves mica	.05 ounce (1.4 grams)

Prepare as directed in the My 'd Azure Lipstick Color Grind recipe.

Umber Penny Lipstick Color Grind

A dark, coppery, rusty red with a satin sheen. It's not too glittery for day wear. This recipe makes .3 ounce (8.5 grams) color grind.

Umber mica	.2 ounce (5.7 grams)
Deep Russet mica	.1 ounce (2.8 grams)

Prepare as directed in the My 'd Azure Lipstick Color Grind recipe.

Nudes

There are times when you only want a hint of color, and that's when the nude category comes in. These barely there colors add just the right touch for that occasion.

Nude Sparks Lipstick Color Grind

A medium-light nude with a small sparkle—just a little touch to make your lips look moist. This recipe makes .45 ounce (12.8 grams) color grind.

Sparkle Rose mica	.15 ounce (4.3 grams)
Aladdin's Lamp mica	.05 ounce (1.4 grams)
Pearl White mica	.05 ounce (1.4 grams)
Butter Yellow mica	.1 ounce (2.8 grams)
Apricot mica	.1 ounce (2.8 grams)

Prepare as directed in the My 'd Azure Lipstick Color Grind recipe.

Nude Model Lipstick Color Grind

A light nude with a touch of pink and a satin sheen. This recipe makes .3 ounce (8.5 grams) color grind.

Artisan Coral mica	.05 ounce (1.4 grams)
Pearl White or White mica	.1 ounce (2.8 grams)
TKB Trading Matte Texture Base	1 Tad

Prepare as directed in the My 'd Azure Lipstick Color Grind recipe.

Flirtatious Bride Lipstick Color Grind

The lightest nude with only a hint of pink and satin sheen. This recipe makes .3 ounce (8.5 grams) color grind.

Ivory Lace mica	.1 ounce (2.8 grams)
Angel Wings mica	.1 ounce (2.8 grams)
Super Pearl mica	1 Tad

Prepare as directed in the My 'd Azure Lipstick Color Grind recipe.

Oranges

Get out your sunglasses for this section because these color grinds are bright and fiery! If you love the orange tones, I'm sure you'll have fun with these grinds.

Autumn Orange Lipstick Color Grind

The color of autumn leaves with a fiery spark. This recipe makes .3 ounce (8.5 grams) color grind.

Orange oxide	.05 ounce (1.4 grams)
Umber mica	.15 ounce (4.3 grams)
Extra Bright White mica	.05 ounce (1.4 grams)
Red oxide	1 Pinch

Prepare as directed in the My 'd Azure Lipstick Color Grind recipe.

Orange Sorbet Lipstick Color Grind

A bright coral/orange with lots of sparkle. This recipe makes .3 ounce (8.5 grams) color grind.

Pink Coral mica	.2 ounce (5.7 grams)
Red #170 or red oxide	1 Dash

Prepare as directed in the My 'd Azure Lipstick Color Grind recipe.

Peaches

The peach tones go with so many skin tones and hair colors that they're very important to include in any cosmetic line. These lovely colors work perfectly for home or office and even evening wear.

Sizzling Lipstick Color Grind

A soft peachy orange with a touch of pink and sparkle. This recipe makes .3 ounce (8.5 grams) color grind.

Sparkling Rose mica	.05 ounce (1.4 grams)
Pink Coral mica	.1 ounce (2.8 grams)
Apricot mica	.1 ounce (2.8 grams)
Antique Copper mica	1 Tad

Prepare as directed in the My 'd Azure Lipstick Color Grind recipe.

Peaches 'N' Brown Sugar Lipstick Color Grind

A peachy brown, not too dark and not too brown, but a warm color. This recipe makes .3 ounce (8.5 grams) color grind.

Aladdin's Lamp mica	.1 ounce (2.8 grams)
Bronze Fine mica	.1 ounce (2.8 grams)
TKB Trading Matte Texture Base	.1 ounce (2.8 grams)

Prepare as directed in the My 'd Azure Lipstick Color Grind recipe.

Pinks

Pinks are so perfect for day or night. They reflect a natural look while making the lips look soft, moist, and kissable.

Sweet Kisses Lipstick Color Grind

A very light pink with a slight blue undertone. This recipe makes .3 ounce (8.5 grams) color grind.

Ultramarine Ink mica	.05 ounce (1.4 grams)
Angel Wings mica	.25 ounce (7.1 grams)

Prepare as directed in the My 'd Azure Lipstick Color Grind recipe.

Strawberry Pearls Lipstick Color Grind

A medium strawberry pink with sparkle. This recipe makes .3 ounce (8.5 grams) color grind.

Strawberry Pop mica	.1 ounce (2.8 grams)
Pearl White mica	.2 ounce (5.7 grams)

Prepare as directed in the My 'd Azure Lipstick Color Grind recipe.

Pink Taffy Lipstick Color Grind

A medium bright iridescent pink with a sparkle. This recipe makes .2 ounce (5.7 grams) color grind.

Be My Valentine mica	.15 ounce (4.3 grams)
Cloisonne Red mica	.05 ounce (1.4 grams)

Prepare as directed in the My 'd Azure Lipstick Color Grind recipe.

Spun Sugar Lipstick Color Grind

A medium pink with a slight blue undertone and sparkle. This recipe makes .2 ounce (5.7 grams) color grind.

Bronze Fine mica	.1 ounce (2.8 grams)
Sparkling Rose mica	.1 ounce (2.8 grams)

Prepare as directed in the My 'd Azure Lipstick Color Grind recipe.

Sweetheart Pink Lipstick Color Grind

A barely there pink with a touch of beige—very light and very neutral. This recipe makes .26 ounce (7.4 grams) color grind.

Blush Beige mica	.1 ounce (2.8 grams)
Cotton Candy mica	.1 ounce (2.8 grams)
Tibetan Ochre mica	.05 ounce (1.4 grams)
TKB Trading Matte Texture Base	1 Tad

Prepare as directed in the My 'd Azure Lipstick Color Grind recipe.

Plums

Many people love plum-colored lipsticks. Here are some grinds we're sure you'll enjoy using.

In the Plum Lipstick Color Grind

A medium plum with strong pink highlights. This isn't sparkly but has a shine and a sheen. This recipe makes .3 ounce (8.5 grams) color grind.

Sparkling Rose mica	.1 ounce (2.8 grams)
Magnesium Violet mica	.1 ounce (2.8 grams)
Oriental Beige mica	.1 ounce (2.8 grams)

Prepare as directed in the My 'd Azure Lipstick Color Grind recipe.

Plum Berries Lipstick Color Grind

A dark and deep reddish-plum with a satin sheen. Great for evening wear but also during the day for special outings. This recipe makes .25 ounce (7.1 grams) color grind.

Magnesium Violet mica	.1 ounce (2.8 grams)
Antique Copper mica	.1 ounce (2.8 grams)
Colorona Russet mica	.05 ounce (1.4 grams)

Prepare as directed in the My 'd Azure Lipstick Color Grind recipe.

Reds

Who doesn't love red lipstick? For day or evening, nothing pulls everything together like red lips. This section offers several grinds we hope you'll enjoy making—and wearing.

Red Spiced Cinnamon Lipstick Color Grind

A dark and deep reddish-brown with a light sparkle. Wearable during the day or at night, this is a very versatile color for just about everyone. This recipe makes .35 ounce (9.9 grams) color grind.

Red oxide	.05 ounce (1.4 grams)
Hot Momma mica	.1 ounce (2.8 grams)
Antique Copper mica	.1 ounce (2.8 grams)
Burning Leaves mica	.1 ounce (2.8 grams)

Prepare as directed in the My 'd Azure Lipstick Color Grind recipe.

Incurable Romantic Lipstick Color Grind

A deep and sexy red with a satin sheen. This is the perfect knock-'em-dead red for evening or maybe even a business meeting. This recipe makes .4 ounce (11.3 grams) color grind.

Red #170	.2 ounce (5.7 grams)
Crucible Red mica	.2 ounce (5.7 grams)

Prepare as directed in the My 'd Azure Lipstick Color Grind recipe.

Deep Chestnut Lipstick Color Grind

The name pretty well describes this rich red-brown color. This color grind is more of a brown than a red tone, and the Burning Leaves mica sets it on fire with sparkle. This recipe makes .25 ounce (7.1 grams) color grind.

Red oxide—blue shade	.1 ounce (2.8 grams)
Antique Copper mica	.1 ounce (2.8 grams)
Burning Leaves mica	.05 ounce (1.4 grams)

Prepare as directed in the My 'd Azure Lipstick Color Grind recipe.

Delicious Intentions Lipstick Color Grind

A deep bluish-red with a satin sheen and a slight sparkle. This is a sexy and seductive rich red—only wear it when you have delicious intentions! This recipe makes .2 ounce (8.5 grams) color grind.

Glitter Bordeaux mica	.1 ounce (2.8 grams)
Queen Kathryn mica	.05 ounce (1.4 grams)
Crucible Red mica	.05 ounce (1.4 grams)
Red oxide	1 Drop

Prepare as directed in the My 'd Azure Lipstick Color Grind recipe.

Making Lipstick Pencils

If you love to line your lips before you put on lipstick, this section is for you. Lining your lips not only helps define your lips but also keeps your lipstick from bleeding or going where it shouldn't go.

Our lipstick pencils are made just like our eyeliner pencils. Follow these recipes and instructions, and refer to the photographs in Chapter 10's "Making Eyeliners" section for clarification on how to fill your pencils.

When applying your makeup, use the same color grind, or one that complements it, for your lip pencil as your lipstick.

Here's what you need to make lipstick pencils:

- Scale

- Small saucepan or heat-resistant glass measuring cup

- Spoons

- 3mm pipettes

- Hollow pencils

- Syringe, with no needle

- Cup

- Stove or microwave

Lip Liner Pencil Base

Recently I went into a department store and was shocked at the prices for lip liner and eyeliner pencils. You can make these pencils for a tiny fraction of what stores charge. They're easy and only take a few minutes to make. We make lip liner pencils using the same method as used for eyeliner pencils. The same hollow pencils are used, too. You can match your lipstick perfectly by using the same color grind to make the lip liner pencil. I've found that the longer they're allowed to cure, the better they are. I give mine a month. This recipe makes 1 ounce (28.4 grams), or enough base to fill 8 pencils.

Beeswax	.1 ounce (2.8 grams)
Candelilla wax	.2 ounce (5.7 grams)
Palm kernel stearin	.2 ounce (5.7 grams)
Jojoba oil	.2 ounce (5.7 grams)
Castor oil	.2 ounce (5.7 grams)
Preservative	.11 ounce (3.1 grams)
Color grind	.1 ounce (2.8 grams)

1. Place a small container on the scale, and push the tare button to zero out the weight of the container. Weigh each of the waxes, and place them in the saucepan or heat-resistant glass cup. Weigh the rest of the ingredients except the color grind. Place them in the saucepan or cup.

2. Heat over low heat or in the microwave on half power until all the waxes have melted completely.

3. While the waxes are melting, weigh your color grind and have it ready to add to the wax mixture. Remember to push the tare button before weighing the color grind.

4. When the waxes are melted, stir in the color grind until the grind has dissolved completely. At this time you may need to reheat the mixture just a little.

5. Draw up the liquid into the syringe. While holding the pencil with one end flat against the counter, fill the other end with the liquid lip liner. The mixture needs to be hot enough to flow easily down the hollow pencil shaft. When it's filled to the top, set the pencil upright in a cup to cool. Continue filling your pencils, reheating when necessary.

6. Set the pencils in an out-of-the-way place so they can cure for a few days before you sharpen them. Store any leftover base in a zipper-lock bag for later use.

The Least You Need to Know

- Everyone will love the lip balms you make from this chapter, so make extra so you can share!
- Be sure you have the right kind of scale for the color grinds. The scale will need to weigh grams to the 100th.
- All the micas and oxides are given by their actual name so you will know which ones to buy and be able to make the exact grinds in this chapter.

For the Fellas and Beyond

We've given you tons of recipes and DIY information in the preceding three parts, but we're not done yet! In Part 4, we remember the guys in your life (who might be feeling a little left out when they see how much fun you're having and how lovely you look!). So Part 4 begins with a chapter for all things male so you can pamper him. And last but definitely not least, check out our bits and pieces chapter. It's chock-full of lots of fun recipes that didn't fit elsewhere.

One thing we know for sure: you will love making all kinds of natural and earth-friendly beauty products. (And if that isn't enough to keep you busy, check out our companion book, *The Complete Idiot's Guide to Making Natural Soaps*, too!)

For the Guys

In This Chapter

- After-shave lotions or splashes for your fella
- Manly moisturizers, facials, and colognes
- Anti-aging recipes—men need them, too!

Men today aren't so opposed to using lotions and toners as their counterparts were 20 years ago. Men also need to use moisturizers, anti-aging serums, facials, and after-bath powders. Whatever manly product you're looking for, you've come to the right chapter.

Not all the recipes will be simple, however. Some are pretty complicated, but never fear: we walk you through each step. And trust us: the results are worth it—especially when the men in your life realize how much work you put in for them! And they'll love being pampered once they get past the "I'm a man, and we don't do that stuff" thing. If they balk, just tell them to man up and do it.

Okay, guys. It's time to cowboy up and start taking better care of your skin to keep the cowgirls happy.

The Basics of Making Manly Products

First things first: let's talk about scent. When scenting products for guys, you'll want to use manly fragrance oils or a blend of essential oils suitable for the fellas.

Balsam of Peru is a wonderful and manly essential oil, but use only a few drops at a time. It can make just about any fragrance oil manly. Try blending it with a floral fragrance oil to give the fragrance oil a new twist. Or try mixing a couple drops of balsam of Peru with sandalwood fragrance oil. Lemongrass essential oil is great for closing and shrinking pores. Blend the lemongrass essential oil with lime essential oil for a fresh citrus scent. Even though lavender essential oil is very antiseptic, we doubt you'll want your husband/partner to smell like your grandmother! Instead, you can blend the lavender with patchouli and still have the antiseptic benefits. Try your hand at blending the essential oils a few drops at a time, and create a nice-smelling, manly blend that will also have skin-loving benefits.

Here's what you need to create the products in this chapter for the men in your life:

- Scales
- Stove
- Stainless-steel pot
- Immersion blender
- Stainless-steel saucepan
- Glass, stainless-steel, or plastic bowls
- Glass cup
- Thermometer
- Spatulas and spoons
- Jars and bottles

IN THE MIRROR

As noted earlier, we don't include the amount of preservative or scent as part of the 100 percent makeup of these recipes. Scent is optional, and the amount of preservative depends on the type and brand of preservative you use. (See Appendix E.) I like to use Optiphen Plus. It's paraben- and formaldehyde-free. Use 1 percent of the total weight of the product you're making.

Fragrance Blends for Men

Alex Crow, "the happy blender," created these for-men-only blends for the Apples, Woods and Berries website and has graciously allowed us to include them in this book. (If you like these, be sure to look for Alex's online e-book, *The Alchemy of Fragrance Blending*.)

Each blend is written in "parts" so you can make any amount of a blend you need, and it will come out perfect every time. A "part" can be anything you want or need it to be, from 1 ounce to 16 ounces.

His Texas Waltz Fragrance Blend

With Cherokee Creek's soft woodsy and earthy notes, this blend kicks up its heels with a spicy touch of pepperberry.

    1 part Cherokee Creek
    1 part pepperberry

His Cowboy Two-Step Fragrance Blend

The always-classic Irish green tweed is even sexier with the addition of the sweet woods and musk of Hardwood Musk.

    2 parts Hardwood Musk
    1 part Irish green tweed

His Tropical Spice Fragrance Blend

Sweet berries soften the tart pineapple and lush mango. The spicy pepper of pepperberry spurs the blend into a sensation!

    1 part pepperberry
    1 part pineapple mango

His Blackberry Tweed Fragrance Blend

The green herbaceous and woody notes of the Irish green tweed give a sexy masculine twist to the fruity fragrance of blackberry apple.

    2 parts blackberry apple
    1 part Irish green tweed

IN THE MIRROR

You can also use these blends when making cologne. To make a men's cologne, use 80 percent perfumer's alcohol and 20 percent fragrance or essential oil.

His Handsome and Distinguished Fragrance Blend

Masculine and sexy, Cowboy Campfire blends with the soft earthy sandalwood and joins the woodsiness of Hardwood Musk to yield a very handsome and distinguished one-of-a-kind fragrance.

4 parts Cowboy Campfire

1 part Hardwood Musk

1 part sandalwood

Making Men's Shaving Cream

Nearly every man uses shaving cream, so why not make him an all-natural version? The following recipe will not only offer slip for shaving but also all the skin-softening benefits of a cream.

If you're interested in making him a shaving soap, please check out our companion book, *The Complete Idiot's Guide to Making Natural Soaps.*

IN THE MIRROR

By the time of the Crusades, fragrance, aromas, and spices were being used to mask body odor. In 1709, the first "cologne" was created. More than 179 years later, in 1888, deodorant was invented in the United States. Then in 1952, roll-on deodorant was introduced to the market. The first aerosol spray deodorant appeared in 1965.

His Shaving Cream

With this recipe, you'll first make a very thick cream. After the cream has cooled and thickened overnight—yep, this is a 2-day recipe—you'll add liquids and additives to create a skin-soothing and -lubricating shaving cream. It has the best of both a shaving soap and a moisturizer. This original recipe was posted on a Yahoo! soap group, but we made a few changes in our version. This recipe can be doubled if you desire. Please read these instructions all the way through before you begin. This recipe makes 1 (8-ounce; 226.8-gram) or 2 (4-ounce; 113.4-gram) sterile jar(s).

Part 1:

Distilled water	2.8 ounces (79.4 grams)
Emulsifying wax	.3 ounce (8.5 grams)
Sweet almond oil	.5 ounce (14.2 grams)

Follow directions for making the Thick and Luscious Body Butter in Chapter 12.

Part 2:

Aloe vera juice	2 ounces (56.7 grams)
Xanthan gum or HEC (Xanthan is best.)	.25 ounce (7.1 grams)
Bentonite clay	.3 ounce (8.5 grams)
Grapeseed oil	.3 ounce (8.5 grams)
Dimethicone	.5 ounce (14.2 grams)
Witch hazel	1 ounce (28.4 grams)
Preservative	(see manufacturer's recommendation)
Essential oil blend (your choice)	.1 ounce (2.8 grams)

1. Put a small bowl on your scale, push the tare button, and weigh the aloe vera juice.

2. Pour the aloe vera juice into a small saucepan, and set it over low heat. When it has warmed to 110°F, remove from heat.

3. While the juice is warming, put another small bowl on the scale, push the tare button, and weigh the xanthan gum and bentonite clay. Place each into two small bowls.

4. Put a bowl on the scales, and again push the tare button. Weigh the grapeseed oil and the dimethicone. Set them aside for now.

5. After the aloe vera has warmed, remove it from heat. Remove a small amount of the warm aloe vera juice, and stir it into the xanthan. Then do the same with the clay to make a wet paste.

6. Add both xanthan and clay mixtures to the warmed aloe vera juice, and stir until everything is well incorporated. It should start to become a nice, thick gel.

7. Add the witch hazel, and the thick cream from part 1 to the aloe vera mixture. Stir well using a whisk or spoon.

8. Add the grapeseed oil and the dimethicone, including the preservative and scent, and stir until it's all well incorporated.

9. Bottle in a pump or squeeze bottle.

IN THE MIRROR

You can use HEC, hydroxyethylcellulose, in this recipe. It's made from cellulose or xanthan gum and is used for thickening.

Making After-Shave Splash

After-shave splashes are very easy to make. Because the skin can become so irritated after shaving, it needs to be soothed and the pores closed. That's where after-shave splashes come in. These splashes are cold made, which means no heat is applied. Just weigh the ingredients, mix, and bottle. It's that simple!

Here's what you need to make after-shave splashes:

- Scale

- Small pitcher

- 1 small bowl and 1 large bowl

- Spoon

- Sterile bottle

IN THE MIRROR

Lemongrass essential oil helps close and tighten pores, so it's an excellent choice to use in a scent blend for after-shave splashes.

His Old Lime After-Shave Splash

Alcohol is not used in this recipe, so this splash is well suited for men who have sensitive skin. It also contains edelweiss extract, which is anti-inflammatory, antioxidant, anti-aging, and antifungal; it also fights bacteria. This recipe makes 1 (16-ounce; 453.6-gram) or 2 (8-ounce; 226.8-gram) sterile bottle(s).

Aloe vera juice	9 ounces (255.1 grams)
Edelweiss extract	.8 ounce (22.7 grams)
Witch hazel	6.1 ounces (172.9 grams)
Lime essential oil	.1 ounce (2.8 grams)
Preservative	(see manufacturer's recommendation)

1. Put a small pitcher or bowl on your scale, and push the tare button. Weigh the aloe vera juice. Set it aside for a minute.

2. Put a small bowl on the scale, and push the tare button. Weigh the edelweiss extract. Add it to the aloe vera juice, and stir until it's dissolved.

3. Put a bowl on your scale, and push the tare button. Weigh the witch hazel, and add it to the aloe vera mixture. Repeat for the lime essential oil and the preservative.

4. Mix together well, and bottle in a sterile bottle(s).

His Embracing After-Shave Splash

This recipe is for the man who wants alcohol in his after-shave splash. This is a basic recipe you can add extra ingredients to and make it your own. You can use distilled water in place of aloe vera juice if you want, and you can double this recipe as many times as you like. This recipe makes 1 (8-ounce; 226.8-gram) or 2 (4-ounce; 113.4-gram) sterile bottle(s).

Aloe vera juice	5 ounces (141.7 grams)
Witch hazel	2.5 ounces (70.9 grams)
Alcohol	.5 ounce (14.2 grams)
Fragrance oil blend or essential oil	.8 ounce (22.7 grams)
Preservative	(see manufacturer's recommendation)

Prepare as directed in the His Old Lime After-Shave Splash recipe.

SAFETY FIRST

When using essential oils in a recipe, don't use more than 2.5 percent of the total weight of the mixture. Essential oils are very strong and can irritate the skin. For fragrance oils, don't use more than 3 percent. More than that can cause skin irritation.

Making After-Shave Lotion

After shaving, men need to use a good after-shave splash or lotion. In several of these recipes, we've used aloe vera gel or juice in place of water to add skin-soothing benefits. And after-shave lotion makes a great carrier for the anti-aging and antiwrinkle additives available today.

Here's what you need to make after-shave lotion:

- Stove
- Medium stainless-steel saucepan
- Scale
- Thermometer
- Small glass or plastic bowls
- Immersion blender
- Spoons
- Small glass or stainless-steel cup

His Cowboy Two-Step After-Shave Lotion

Fragrance blend created and named by Alex Crow.

Men love anti-aging products as much as women do. This recipe uses a four-ingredient blend of anti-aging additives that really works! I use them in creams for women, too. You can find these ingredients online at Lotioncrafter (lotioncrafter.com). This recipe makes 1 (16-ounce; 453.6-gram) or 2 (8-ounce; 226.8-gram) sterile bottle(s) or jar(s).

Sweet almond oil	2.4 ounces (68 grams)
Meadowfoam seed oil	2 ounces (56.7 grams)
Emulsifying wax	1.1 ounces (31.2 grams)
Aloe vera juice	7 ounces (198.4 grams)

When the lotion has cooled down to 104°F, add:

Lotioncrafter Wrinkle Defense Complex	1.4 ounces (39.7 grams)
Hyaluronic acid (anti-aging)	.1 ounce (2.8 grams)
Decorinyl (anti-aging)	.5 ounce (14.2 grams)

Edelweiss extract	.5 ounce (14.2 grams)
Distilled water	1 ounce (28.4 grams)
Preservative	(see manufacturer's recommendation)
Fragrance blend	.2 ounce (5.7 grams)

Fragrance blend:

Hardwood musk	.15 ounce (4.3 grams)
Irish green tweed	.05 ounce (1.4 grams)

1. Place a bowl on the scale, and push the tare button. Weigh your first oil, and pour it into the saucepan. Put the bowl back on the scale, push the tare button, and continue weighing the oils and emulsifying wax. Pour them into the saucepan. Place the pan over low heat, and let the wax completely melt.

2. Place a fresh bowl on the scale, and push the tare button. Weigh the aloe vera juice. Pour into a separate saucepan, and set it over low heat.

3. Put a fresh small bowl on the scale, and push the tare button. Weigh the Lotioncrafter Wrinkle Defense Complex, hyaluronic acid, decorinyl, and edelweiss extract predissolved in distilled water.

4. In separate bowls, weigh the preservative and fragrance blend. Set aside.

5. Add the warmed aloe to the oil mixture, and use an immersion blender to bring the oils, wax, and water together to form a good emulsion. Remove from heat.

6. When mixture has cooled to 110°F, add the preservative and fragrance blend as well. Let it continue to cool to 104°F and add Wrinkle Defense Complex, hyaluronic acid, decorinyl, and edelweiss extract. Again use the immersion blender to incorporate all the ingredients. At this time, you can also add a skin-safe colorant. Let cool completely; as the mixture cools, it will thicken into a rich lotion. Package in sterile bottles or jars.

His Essentially After-Shave Lotion

After-shave lotions and splashes are an important step to close the pores and prevent shaving bumps after shaving. In this recipe, we've used a blend of two essential oils that helps close the pores and leaves a nice, citrus scent on his skin. This recipe makes 24 ounces (680.4 grams), or 4 (8-ounce; 226.8-gram) bottles or 8 (4-ounce; 113.4-gram) bottles.

Cocoa butter	.8 ounce (22.7 grams)
Sweet almond oil	2 ounces (56.7 grams)
Meadowfoam seed oil	2 ounces (56.7 grams)
Emulsifying wax	1.2 ounces (34 grams)
Distilled water	8.4 ounces (238.1 grams)
Aloe vera gel	8.4 ounces (238.1 grams)
Preservative	(see manufacturer's recommendation)

Essential oil blend:

Lemon or lime essential oil	.1 ounce (2.8 grams)
Sweet orange essential oil	.1 ounce (2.8 grams)
Clove essential oil	a dash

Or try this:

| Patchouli essential oil | .1 ounce (2.8 grams) |
| Balsam of Peru essential oil | .05 ounce (1.4 grams) |

Prepare as directed in the His Cowboy Two-Step After-Shave Lotion recipe.

Making After-Bath Powders

In addition to making skin feel nice and smooth, after-bath powders keep a man's skin dry and more comfortable. When antiseptic essential oils are used in the mix, the after-bath powder also eliminates any bacteria-caused odors. You can buy fillable shaker containers online. Most are 4 or 5 ounces (113.4 to 141.7 grams).

Here's what you need to make after-bath powders:

- Scale
- Small plastic or glass bowls
- Large plastic or glass bowl
- Spatula or spoon
- Latex gloves
- Shaker containers or airtight container for storage

His Dry and Comfortable After-Bath Powder

Nutrasorb is a natural starch that absorbs oils and moisture and helps in this recipe to keep your man dry and comfortable all day long. This recipe makes 20 ounces (566.9 grams) or 5 (4-ounce; 113.4-gram) shaker containers.

Nutrasorb	8 ounces (226.8 grams)
Baking soda	8 ounces (226.8 grams)
Cornstarch	4 ounces (113.4 grams)
Men's essential oil blend or fragrance oil	.15 ounce (4.3 grams)

1. Place a bowl on your scale, push the tare button, and weigh your first ingredient. Pour that into a large bowl. Repeat until you've weighed all the dry ingredients.

2. With latex gloves on, use your hands to mix the dry ingredients until they're well incorporated.

3. Place a small cup on the scale, push the tare button, and weigh the essential oils.

4. With latex gloves still on, drizzle the essential oil blend into the dry ingredients, and use your hands to work the oils into the dry mixture. Package in a shaker container or an airtight container.

His Deodorizing After-Bath Powder

While leaving his skin cool, dry, and refreshed, this powder also helps keep him smelling nice, thanks to its deodorizing ingredients. This recipe makes 24 ounces (680.4 grams) or 6 (4-ounce; 113.4-gram) shaker containers.

Arrowroot	8 ounces (226.8 grams)
Baking soda	8 ounces (226.8 grams)
Cornstarch	8 ounces (226.8 grams)
Cypress essential oil	.05 ounce (2.5 milliliters)
Rosemary essential oil	.05 ounce (2.5 milliliters)
Sage essential oil	.05 ounce (2.5 milliliters)
Thyme essential oil	.05 ounce (2.5 milliliters)

Prepare as directed in the His Dry and Comfortable After-Bath Powder recipe.

IN THE MIRROR

For centuries, arrowroot has been the main medicine tribal medicine men have used for healing wounds. The native tribes of countries such as Brazil even use arrowroot for wounds made by poisoned arrows and for infections such as gangrene. It's still in use today.

After you have these essentials as a blend, you may also want to add a few drops of other essential or fragrance oils to make a fragrant blend more to your liking.

Making Manly Moisturizers

Using a moisturizer every day helps keep a man's skin looking soft and youthful. Lotions and moisturizers are made the same way, so follow the lotion directions for these recipes.

Here's what you need to make moisturizers for him:

- Stove
- Stainless-steel saucepan
- Scale
- Glass or plastic bowls

- Thermometer
- Immersion blender
- Spatula and spoons
- Bottles

His Mature Skin Facial Moisturizer

Just like women, as a man ages, his skin needs more moisture to keep it soft. This moisturizer is perfect for the mature man's skin needs. This recipe makes 1 (16-ounce; 453.6-gram) or 2 (8-ounce; 226.8-gram) sterile bottles.

Castor oil	1 ounce (28.4 grams)
Meadowfoam seed oil	1 ounce (28.4 grams)
Apricot kernel oil	1.9 ounces (53.9 grams)
Emulsifying wax	.8 ounce (22.7 grams)
Distilled water	8 ounces (226.8 grams)
Aloe vera juice	4 ounces (113.4 grams)
Lemongrass essential oil	.1 ounce (2.8 grams)
Preservative	(see manufacturer's recommendation)

Prepare as directed in the His Cowboy Two-Step After-Shave Lotion recipe.

His Light Facial Moisturizer

This moisturizer offers just a little extra help to keep his skin soft and kissable. Give it to younger men who just want to keep their skin soft and young-looking longer. This recipe makes 1 (16-ounce; 453.6-gram) or 2 (8-ounce; 226.8-gram) sterile bottles.

Avocado oil	1 ounce (28.4 grams)
Grapeseed oil	1 ounce (28.4 grams)
Sweet almond oil	1.2 ounces (34 grams)
Emulsifying wax	.8 ounce (22.7 grams)
Aloe vera juice (or distilled water)	12 ounces (340.2 grams)
Essential or fragrance oil	.2 ounce (5.7 grams)
Preservative	(see manufacturer's recommendation)

Prepare as directed in the His Cowboy Two-Step After-Shave Lotion recipe.

His Light Facial Moisturizer for Acne-Prone Skin

Even young men who have acne-prone skin need a little moisturizer. This is a very light recipe and won't aggravate acne. This recipe makes 1 (16-ounce; 453.6-gram) or 2 (8-ounce; 226.8-gram) sterile bottles.

Meadowfoam seed oil	1.2 ounces (34 grams)
Jojoba oil	2 ounces (56.7 grams)
Emulsifying wax	.8 ounce (22.7 grams)
Aloe vera juice (or distilled water)	12 ounces (340.2 grams)
Calendula essential oil	.2 ounce (5.7 grams)
Lemongrass essential oil	.1 ounce (2.8 grams)
Tangerine essential oil	.1 ounce (2.8 grams)

Prepare as directed in the His Cowboy Two-Step After-Shave Lotion recipe.

Making Exfoliants for Men

Just like women, men have dead skin, too! We created these "manly" exfoliants so our men can keep their skin in great health and looking good. A man should use an exfoliant at least once a week.

Many people love to use sea salt in their *exfoliants,* but sea salt is too rough on the skin and actually tears the delicate tissues. Sugar eats bacteria, so using sugar is a great way to clear up the skin while also removing dead skin cells.

BEAUTY BIT

An **exfoliant** helps remove the oldest, dead skin cells that lie on the top layer of the skin.

To use exfoliants, wet his face, scoop out about 1 tablespoon (14.8 milliliters), and rub all over his face in circular motions. Use more scrub if needed to cover his entire face. Rinse with warm water, and pat dry.

Here's what you need to make exfoliants:

- Food processor
- Scale
- Plastic or glass bowls
- Spatula or spoon
- 2-ounce jar

His Oily Skin Exfoliant

For men who have oily skin and are prone to breakouts, this recipe is for you. The sugar eats the bacteria, and the jojoba oil won't aggravate pimples. This recipe can be doubled as many times as you want. This recipe makes 1 (2-ounce; 56.7-gram) sterile jar.

Brown sugar	1 ounce (28.4 grams)
Jojoba oil	.5 ounce (14.2 grams)
Finely ground *apricot kernel meal*	.5 ounce (14.2 grams)
Preservative	(see manufacturer's recommendation)

1. Place the bowl on the scale, and push the tare button. Weigh all the ingredients one at a time, and place in the bowl of a food processor.

2. Grind for at least 1 minute, and package in a sterile jar.

His Normal and Dry Skin Exfoliant

This is a great exfoliant for most types of skin and ages. This recipe can be doubled as many times as you want. This recipe makes 1 (2-ounce; 56.7-gram) sterile jar.

Finely ground oatmeal	1 ounce (28.4 grams)
Jojoba beads	.5 ounce (14.2 grams)
Sweet almond oil	.5 ounce (14.2 grams)
Preservative	(see manufacturer's recommendation)

Prepare as directed in the His Oily Skin Exfoliant recipe.

Making Men's Skin-Tightening Masks

Men need to use masks, too. After all, they have the same pollutants in their skin as women do. Using a mask once a week helps keep a man's skin tight, his pores clean, and his skin toxin- and pollutant-free.

To use these masks, remove about 1 tablespoon (14.8 milliliters) and place in your hand. Add enough distilled water to the powder to make a medium paste—thin enough to spread but not so thin it drips. Spread evenly over his face, avoiding his eye area. Let dry for about 20 minutes. Have him sit back and relax and enjoy his "me" time. Rinse off with warm water and pat dry. Follow mask with a moisturizer.

Here's what you need to make skin-tightening masks:

- Coffee grinder or small food processor
- Scale
- Bowls
- Spatula or spoon
- Sterile jar or airtight container for storage

His Skin-Tightening and Moisturizing Mask

This mask is great for any skin type. It not only pulls out all the toxins and pollution but also moisturizes his skin. This recipe makes 1 (2-ounce; 56.7-gram) sterile jar.

White kaolin clay	1 ounce (28.4 grams)
Avocado oil	1 ounce (28.4 grams)
Honeyquat	.1 ounce (2.8 grams)
Lavender essential oil	6 drops
Preservative	(see manufacturer's recommendation)

1. Place a container on the scale, and push the tare button. Weigh each ingredient, and place it in the bowl of your coffee grinder.

2. Grind the ingredients together for 1 minute, stir ingredients around in bowl, and grind for another minute. If you don't have a coffee grinder, you can use a mortar and pestle.

3. Pour mask into a sterile jar until ready to use.

How to use this mask:

1. Remove 1 tablespoon (14.8 milliliters) mask, and mix it with enough water to make a nice spreadable paste.

2. Smooth the mask over your face and throat, avoiding your eye area.

3. Relax with a book or magazine while your mask dries.

4. Rinse off with warm water, and pat face dry with a soft towel.

5. Follow with a pore-closing toner.

His Exfoliant and Cleansing Mask

Men remove a lot of their dead skin cells when they shave, but this mask gets the cells his razor doesn't while it also deep-cleans and draws out the pollutants and toxins. This recipe makes 6 ounces (170.1 grams) or 3 (2-ounce; 56.7-gram) sterile jars.

Kaolin clay (pink, red, black, or yellow)	4 ounces (113.4 grams)
Finely ground oatmeal	2 ounces (56.7 grams)

Prepare as directed in the His Skin-Tightening and Moisturizing Mask recipe.

Making Foot-Care Products for Him

Hey guys! You need to take care of those feet! It is *not* romantic when your feet feel like sandpaper (or your toenails are so long they're like claws)! So do yourself and those around you a favor and care of your feet, whether they're seriously dry or they're … well … not-so-pleasant-smelling.

Here's what you need to make men's foot-care products:

- Stove
- Scale
- Immersion blender
- Medium stainless-steel saucepan
- Thermometer
- Small plastic or glass bowls
- Large plastic or stainless-steel bowl
- Spatula and spoons
- Small glass or stainless-steel cup
- Sterile jar(s)

His Exfoliating Foot Cream

This cream removes dead skin while it softens the skin on the feet. You'll actually see the little balls of dead skin roll off your feet as you rub in this cream. Be sure to rinse off your feet afterward to remove all the little dead-skin balls. You can double this recipe as many times as you like. This recipe makes 16 ounces (453.6 grams).

Grapeseed oil	1 ounce (28.4 grams)
Sweet almond oil	1 ounce (28.4 grams)
Jojoba beads	1 ounce (28.4 grams)
Emulsifying wax	1 ounce (28.4 grams)
Distilled water	12 ounces (340.2 grams)
Peppermint essential oil	.1 ounce (2.8 grams)
Preservative	(see manufacturer's recommendation)

1. Prepare as directed in the His Cowboy Two-Step After-Shave Lotion recipe, and let cool completely.

2. To use, rub feet with cream. Keep rubbing while it rolls off the dead skin—you'll actually see little bits of dead skin flake off as you rub. Rinse feet afterward.

IN THE MIRROR

This exfoliant is great for women's feet, too. Why not treat her to a foot rub and exfoliant after she's had a long day?

His Stinky Feet Lotion

Let's face it, feet stink. They sweat in our shoes, and bacteria grow, causing foot odor. Use this cream every morning, and your feet won't have a foul odor at the end of the day when you take off your shoes. Women can use this lotion, too! It's not just for men. You can double this recipe as many times as you like to make the batch size you want. This recipe makes 24 ounces (680.4 grams), 3 (8-ounce; 226.8-gram) sterile bottles, or 6 (4-ounce; 113.4-gram) sterile bottles.

Sweet almond oil	2 ounces (56.7 grams)
Grapeseed oil (or your choice)	2 ounces (56.7 grams)
Cocoa butter	.6 ounce (17 grams)
Emulsifying wax	1.5 ounces (42.5 grams)
Distilled water	10.8 ounces (306.2 grams)
Aloe vera juice	6 ounces (170.1 grams)
Nutrasorb	1 ounce (28.4 grams)
Essential oil blend	.5 ounce (14.2 grams)
Preservative	(see manufacturer's recommendation)

To make the essential oil blend, use equal parts (2.8 grams) of the following to make .5 ounce:

Basil essential oil	Lavender essential oil
Chamomile essential oil	Peppermint essential oil
Eucalyptus essential oil	

Prepare as directed in the His Cowboy Two-Step After-Shave Lotion recipe, and pour into sterile bottles.

PRETTY POINTER

To add the Nutrasorb without it clumping, mix it with a little of the aloe vera juice before adding the Nutrasorb to the mixture.

His Stinky Feet Powder

You can achieve the same results as the His Stinky Feet Lotion in a powder form. Use the powder every morning, just like the lotion, to keep your feet dry and odor-free all day. No longer will you be embarrassed when you remove your shoes. This recipe makes 24 ounces (680.4 grams) or 6 (4-ounce; 113.4-gram) shaker containers.

Skin Flo or Nutrasorb	8 ounces (226.8 grams)
Cornstarch	8 ounces (226.8 grams)
Baking soda	4 ounces (113.4 grams)
Arrowroot	4 ounces (113.4 grams)
Essential oil blend	.5 ounce (2.5 milliliters)
Preservative	(see manufacturer's recommendation)

To make the essential oil blend, use equal parts (2.8 grams) of the following to make .5 ounce:

Basil essential oil	Lavender essential oil
Chamomile essential oil	Peppermint essential oil
Eucalyptus essential oil	

1. In a jar with a screw-on lid, mix together all the dry ingredients. Put the lid on, and shake well.

2. Drizzle the essential oil blend and preservative into the jar a little at a time. Replace the lid, shake like crazy, and drizzle in some more. Repeat until all the essential oil blend is well incorporated.

3. Dust feet with powder every morning. Dust the insides of your shoes, too, for extra coverage.

BEAUTY BIT

Skin Flo, also called Dry Flo, reduces the greasy or oily feeling left on the skin from lotions, creams, and other skin care products. It's made from natural starch. A similar product, Nutrasorb, does the same thing.

His Peppermint Foot Cream

At the end of the day, this cream will relax and rejuvenate his feet. This recipe makes 16 ounces (453.6 grams), 2 (8-ounce; 226.8-gram) sterile jars, or 4 (4-ounce; 113.4-gram) sterile jars.

Cocoa butter	2.4 ounces (68 grams)
Grapeseed oil	2.4 ounces (68 grams)
Sweet almond oil	1.9 ounces (53.9 grams)
Emulsifying wax	.8 ounce (22.7 grams)
Stearic acid	.5 ounce (14.2 grams)
Distilled water	8 ounces (226.8 grams)
Peppermint essential oil	.3 ounce (8.5 grams)
Preservative	.16 ounce (4.5 grams)

Prepare as directed in the His Cowboy Two-Step After-Shave Lotion recipe.

His Seriously Dry and Cracked Foot Mask

This is a very hydrating foot mask that soothes and helps heal dry and chapped skin. This recipe makes 16 ounces (453.6 grams), 2 (8-ounce; 226.8-gram) sterile jars, or 4 (4-ounce; 113.4-gram) sterile jars.

Lanolin	4 ounces (113.4 grams)
Sweet almond oil	2 ounces (56.7 grams)
Apricot kernel oil	1 ounce (28.4 grams)
Castor oil	1 ounce (28.4 grams)
Emulsifying wax	1 ounce (28.4 grams)
Stearic acid	.5 ounce (14.2 grams)
Aloe vera juice	6.5 ounces (184.2 grams)
Fragrance or essential oil	.2 ounce (5.7 grams)
Preservative	(see manufacturer's recommendation)

1. Prepare as directed in the His Cowboy Two-Step After-Shave Lotion recipe, and let cool completely.

2. To use, apply a medium-thick coat of mask to your feet. Allow to sit for 30 minutes. Use a tissue to wipe off any excess mask.

His Foot Butter

This wonderful creamy butter makes his feet feel soft and touchable, especially if it's massaged into his feet nightly. This recipe makes 1 (8-ounce; 226.8-gram) or 2 (4-ounce; 113.4-gram) sterile jars.

Shea butter	2 ounces (56.7 grams)
Mango butter	2 ounces (56.7 grams)
Oil (your choice)	4 ounces (113.4 grams)
Preservative	(see manufacturer's recommendation)
Fragrance (optional)	.24 ounce (6.8 grams)

1. Place a bowl on the scale, and push the tare button. Weigh your butters and oils one at a time, and place them in a large bowl.

2. Use an electric mixer and whip the butters, oil, and preservative until it is light and airy.

3. Add the preservative and fragrance, and whip again until well incorporated.

4.. Package in sterile jar(s).

Making Massage Oil for Him

What would a chapter of men's products be without a recipe for massage oil? I doubt there's a man alive who doesn't enjoy getting a massage every once in a while. What better way to pamper your partner than by giving him a massage? Maybe he'll return the favor and give you one, too!

Here's what you need to make his massage oil:

- Bowl
- Scale
- Spoon
- Funnel
- 4-ounce (113.4-gram) bottle

His Massage Oil

Keep the love and romance in your relationship with this delicious massage oil. Just weigh the ingredients, bottle, and use. Warming the oil before giving a massage makes it even more relaxing. This recipe makes 1 (4-ounce; 113.4-gram) sterile bottle.

Macadamia nut oil	1.5 ounces (42.5 grams)
Kukui nut oil or pumpkin seed oil	1 ounce (28.4 grams)
Apricot kernel oil	1 ounce (28.4 grams)
Meadowfoam seed oil	.5 ounce (14.2 grams)

1. Place a bowl on the scale, and push the tare button. Weigh your first oil and set it aside.

2. Place another bowl on the scale, push the tare button, and weigh the next oil, pouring it into the bowl with the first oil. Repeat until all the oils have been weighed. Stir the oils together.

3. Using a funnel, pour the oil mixture into a sterile bottle.

I hope you will find a lot of recipes in this chapter with which to pamper the men in your life!

The Least Need to Know

- Knowing what skin types and needs your man has helps you pick the right recipe or formula for him.
- You can help that teenage boy with his acne and teach him how he needs to take care of his skin by making him personalized manly products.
- Does your man have rough feet? There's a recipe or two here to fix that problem!
- Get out the rope and handcuffs. You might need them for tying him down while he gets his first facial!

Final Bits and Pieces

In This Chapter

- Matching your nail polish to your lipstick
- Fun, glittery items for teens and tweens
- Hand sanitizer, shower sinus tabs, and other useful products
- Special-care items for problem skin

Now for some things that just didn't really fit in any of the other chapters. This is our this-and-that, odds-and-ends, bits-and-pieces chapter.

Home-crafters have been making many of these products for years and years, and not all of these recipes are original to us. But we're sure you'll find lots of recipes in this chapter fun to make and use.

Note that for some of these recipes, you may need to refer to another chapter in the book for directions. When so, we alert you to this fact and tell you which chapter and recipe to turn to.

Those Pearly Whites

In Chapter 1, we discussed the dangers of commercial toothpastes. But there's no need to worry if you make your own dental care products.

Peppermint Toothpowder

This all-natural toothpowder may take a little getting used to, but your teeth and gums will be healthier and whiter when you use it. It's simple to make and use. Just wet your toothbrush, dip it in the powder, and brush as usual. You'll feel the difference from the very first time you use it. This recipe makes .9 ounce (25.5 grams).

Kaolin clay	.3 ounce (8.5 grams)
Bicarbonate soda (baking soda)	.5 ounce (14.2 grams)
Finely ground sea salt	.1 ounce (2.8 grams)
Peppermint or spearmint essential oil	1 to 3 drops
Tea tree essential oil	1 drop

1. Weigh the ingredients on your scale and pour them into the bowl of your grinder or mortar and pestle.

2. Grind the ingredients together for 1 minute.

3. Store toothpowder in an airtight container in between uses.

4. When ready to use, put a little powder in your hand and add a few drops peppermint essential oil and enough tea tree essential oil to the rest of the ingredients to make a paste.

Healthy Gums Toothpowder

If you have gum issues or cavities, this recipe is good to use. Myrrh kills bacteria that attack the teeth and gums. This recipe makes 1 cup (236.6 milliliters).

Finely ground sea salt	½ cup (118.3 milliliters)
Bicarbonate soda (baking soda)	½ cup (118.3 milliliters)
Myrrh	1 teaspoon (4.9 milliliters)
Peppermint essential oil	8 drops
Lemon essential oil	5 drops

Prepare as directed in the Peppermint Toothpowder recipe.

IN THE MIRROR

As noted earlier, we don't include the amount of preservative or scent as part of the 100 percent makeup of these recipes. Scent is optional, and the amount of preservative depends on the type and brand of preservative you use. (See Appendix E.)

Get Your Nails Noticed!

Every beauty book should include a few recipes that help the nails and cuticles. The hand creams and lotions in earlier chapters do help, but sometimes they aren't enough.

Kukui and Shea Cuticle Cream

Give your cuticles some tender loving care with kukui nut oil and shea butter! Just rub a little cream into your cuticles every day to keep them soft and moisturized. Healthy cuticles nourish and grow healthy nails. This recipe makes 2 ounces (56.7 grams).

Shea butter	.6 ounce (17 grams)
Kukui nut oil	.8 ounce (22.7 grams)
White beeswax	.6 ounce (17 grams)
Preservative	(see manufacturer's recommendation)

1. Weigh all the ingredients and place them in a saucepan set over low heat. Heat until all the beeswax has melted. Remove the saucepan from heat.

2. Stir and pour into a small, 2-ounce (56.7-gram) sterile jar. Let stand until completely cool. Screw on lid.

3. To use, rub a little cream into each of your cuticles every day or when they're feeling dry.

Cuticle Oil

This recipe uses more common and less expensive oil but still offers the same benefits, moisturizing and nourishing the cuticles. This recipe makes 2 ounces (56.7 grams).

Shea butter	.4 ounce (11.3 grams)
Jojoba oil	.5 ounce (14.2 grams)
Sweet almond oil	.5 ounce (14.2 grams)
Grapeseed oil	.3 ounce (8.5 grams)
Vitamin E	.3 ounce (8.5 grams)
Preservative	(see manufacturer's recommendation)
Fragrance	2 drops

1. Place a bowl on the scale, and push the tare button. Weigh the shea butter, and place it in a microwavable bowl or in a saucepan over low heat.

2. Using the microwave, heat using low power in short spurts until the butter is almost melted. Remove and stir until all the butter has melted. Do the same if you are using a stove. Remove the butter from the heat while a few unmelted pieces remain, and stir it until it is completely melted.

3. Place a fresh bowl on the scale, and push the tare button. Weigh the other oils, and add them to the melted shea butter. Stir well.

4. Add the vitamin E and preservative. Stir everything together.

5. Pour mixture into a sterilized 2-ounce (56.7-gram) roller ball bottle or a 2-ounce (56.7-gram) bottle with a flip disc top.

Cuticle Stick

I love the convenience of having my cuticle oil in a stick form, and I hope you will, too! You can carry it in your bag and take it with you everywhere. When you want to use it, just apply it to your cuticles and gently rub in. This recipe makes about 5 ounces (141.7 grams), or enough to fill 33 small lip balm tubes.

Soy wax or beeswax	2.25 ounces (63.9 grams)
Shea butter	.5 ounce (14.2 grams)
Mango butter	.5 ounce (14.2 grams)
Sunflower oil	1.5 ounces (42.5 grams)
Vitamin E	.2 ounce (5.7 grams)
Preservative	(see manufacturer's recommendation)

1. Put a bowl on the scale, and push the tare button. Weigh the wax and butters.

2. Put another bowl on the scale, push the tare button, and weigh the remaining ingredients except the preservative. Set them aside for now.

3. Put another small bowl on the scale, push the tare button, and weigh the preservative. Set aside for now.

4. In a saucepan over low heat or in a microwavable container using low heat and short spurts, slowly heat the ingredients until they're almost completely melted.

5. Add the oil and vitamin E. Let it cool down a bit, and add the preservative. Stir everything together, and quickly pour into lip balm tubes.

SAFETY FIRST

Don't forget to label this product! It would be a very yucky-tasting lip balm.

Custom Nail Polish

You can use the mica color grinds in earlier chapters to make awesome nail polish. Buy a bottle of clear nail polish—any brand and type!—and match your lipstick or your eye shadow, or just use one of the pretty color grinds you like. Makes 1 bottle of nail polish.

Store-bought clear nail polish	1 bottle
Color grind from lip or eye chapter	.3 ounce (8.5 grams)

1. Pour a little bit of the polish out into a small bowl, and add the color grind. Stir well, and return mixture to the bottle.

2. Recap and shake thoroughly until color grind is well incorporated in the polish.

3. Test to ensure there's enough color. If not, add a tad more color grind and shake again.

For Teen Girls! And Almost-Teens, Too!

Young girls love to be "sparkly." So here are a few sparkly recipes sure to be a hit with the teens and tweens in your life.

Glitter Gel

This is a fun and simple recipe that's sure to please the preteens, teens, and even post-teens! This recipe can be doubled as many times as needed to make the recipe size you want. This recipe makes 2 ounces (56.7 grams).

Very thick aloe vera gel	2 ounces (56.7 grams)
Very fine glitter or mica	.25 ounce (7.1 grams)
Skin-safe fragrance oil	5 drops
Preservative	(see manufacturer's recommendation)

1. Place a bowl on your scale, and push the tare button. Weigh each ingredient one at a time.

2. Mix all the ingredients together, and stir well.

3. Pour into a sterile 2-ounce (56.7-gram) jar. Screw on the cap.

Glitter Spray

What's more fun than a glitter spray? This spray leaves a light dusting of glitter on the skin. This recipe makes 8 ounces (226.8 grams), or enough to fill 1 (8-ounce; 226.8-gram) fine-mist spray bottle.

Distilled water	3.5 ounces (99.2 grams)
Glycerin	1½ teaspoons (7.4 milliliters)
Very fine glitter or mica	½ teaspoon (2.5 milliliters)
Perfumer's alcohol	4 ounces (113.4 grams)
Fragrance	.2 ounce (5.7 grams)

1. Place a bowl on your scale, and push the tare button. Weigh the distilled water, glycerin, and glitter one at a time.

2. Mix them together, and using a funnel, pour them into a sterile fine-mist spray bottle.

3. Put another bowl on the scale, and push the tare button. Weigh the perfumer's alcohol and fragrance in separate bowls. Set aside for now.

4. Add the fragrance to the bowl with the alcohol. Stir for 1 or 2 minutes. When that's well blended, add to the spray bottle with the other ingredients. Cap and shake well. Shake well again before each use.

Fragrant Body Spray

For this lightly scented body spray, you'll need bottles that have a fine-mist sprayer top. You can even use this same recipe to make spray cologne for guys! This recipe makes 8 ounces (226.8 grams), or 1 (8-ounce; 226.8-gram) fine-mist spray bottle.

Skin-safe fragrance oil	1.6 ounces (45.4 grams)
Cyclomethicone	5.6 ounces (158.8 grams)
Perfumer's alcohol	.8 ounce (22.7 grams)

1. Place a glass measuring cup on your scale, and push the tare button. Weigh the ingredients one at a time, pouring each one into your spray bottle as you weigh them.

2. Screw the spray top on tight, and shake well. Shake well again before each use.

Solid Perfume

This solid perfume is fun. You can toss one pot or jar in your bag and apply it whenever you need a little something extra. You will need 1-ounce (28.4-gram) lip pots or eye shadow jars for these perfumes, and it's best to weigh in grams. You may double this recipe as many times as you like. This recipe makes 1 ounce (28.4 grams).

Oil (your choice)	.5 ounce (14.2 grams)
Beeswax	.36 ounce (10.2 grams)
Skin-safe fragrance or essential oil	.17 ounce (4.7 grams)
Cosmetic glitter (optional)	1 pinch

1. Put a small microwavable container on your scale, and push the tare button to zero out the weight of the container. Weigh the oil and beeswax. Pour into a microwave-safe bowl, and set aside.

2. Put another small container on your scale, and again push the tare button to zero out the weight of this new container. Weigh the scent.

3. Repeat for the glitter.

4. Melt the oil and beeswax in the microwave, on medium heat and in 1-minute spurts. Remove from the microwave, and stir in the scent and glitter.

5. Pour mixture into small sterile lip pots or eye shadow jars.

Zit Be Gone

Get spots or breakouts? This recipe helps clear them up quickly! The roller-ball bottle makes it a snap to apply to each spot, one at a time. This recipe makes 2 ounces (56.7 grams), or enough to fill 1 (2-ounce; 56.7-gram) roller-ball bottle.

Castor oil	.9 ounce (25.5 grams)
Meadowfoam seed oil	.9 ounce (25.5 grams)
Preservative	(see manufacturer's recommendation)
Tea tree essential oil	20 drops
Lavender essential oil	10 drops
Lemongrass essential oil	10 drops

1. Place a glass measuring cup on the scale, and push the tare button. Weigh the first oil. Push the tare button again and weigh the second oil.

2. Mix all weighed ingredients together, and pour into a sterile roller-ball bottle.

3. Using a 3mm pipette, drop the correct number of drops of each essential oil into the roller-ball bottle.

4. Put the roller ball and cap on the bottle, and shake well.

Other Useful Odds and Ends

Now for some other interesting or useful products. Some of these make nice gifts as well.

Pregnant Belly Balm

This balm, packaged in deodorant push-up tubes, is perfect for an expectant mother to carry in her purse and use whenever the need arises or when her skin starts to itch due to stretching. This recipe makes 16 ounces (453.6 grams), or enough for 16 (1-ounce; 28.4-gram) push-up deodorant tubes.

Beeswax pastilles	3.3 ounces (93.6 grams)
Candelilla wax	2 ounces (56.7 grams)
Cocoa butter	2.3 ounces (65.2 grams)
Shea butter	1 ounce (28.4 grams)
Mowrah or mango butter	1 ounce (28.4 grams)
Meadowfoam seed oil	2 ounces (56.7 grams)
Sweet almond oil	1.4 ounces (39.7 grams)
Evening primrose oil	1.5 ounces (42.5 grams)
Avocado oil	1 ounce (28.4 grams)
Pumpkin seed oil	.5 ounce (14.2 grams)
Fragrance or essential oil	.2 ounce (5.7 grams)
Preservative	(see manufacturer's recommendation)

Prepare as directed in the Dry Skin Facial Balm recipe in Chapter 6.

Stretch Mark Oil

The oil is very much like the Pregnant Belly Balm, but it gives more moisturizing. This is best suited to use after your bath. It only takes a minute to completely soak into the skin. This recipe makes 3.5 ounces (99.2 grams).

Fractionated coconut oil	2 ounces (56.7 grams)
Cocoa butter (melted)	1 ounce (28.4 grams)
Apricot kernel oil	.2 ounce (5.7 grams)
Skin-safe fragrance oil	.3 ounce (8.5 grams)

Mix all the ingredients together, and pour into a roller-ball bottle or a spray bottle.

Hand Sanitizer

We all use hand sanitizer, but they're often very drying to the skin so we then find the need to follow it with lotion. This recipe is not drying, and it's just as effective. This recipe makes 2 ounces (56.7 grams).

Very thick aloe vera gel	2 ounces (56.7 grams)
Alcohol (regular)	1 teaspoon (4.9 milliliters)

1. Place a bowl on the scale, and push the tare button. Weigh the aloe vera gel.

2. Add alcohol, and stir well.

3. Using a funnel, pour the mixture into a sterile squeeze bottle or a toggle bottle. Let completely cool.

Fragrance Stones

This recipe is all over the Internet. I don't know who first made these fragrance stones, but I'm glad they did! They are easy and fun to make. You can put them in a bowl and use them as a room freshener or maybe in your drawers with your favorite sweaters—anywhere you want a nice scent. Try not to make the rocks very large. I make mine just a little bigger than pebble size so I can have more rocks.

Flour	1½ cups (354.9 milliliters)
Salt	¼ cup (59.2 milliliters)
Cornstarch	¼ teaspoon (1.2 milliliters)
Fragrance oil	1 tablespoon (14.8 milliliters)
Coloring	(see manufacturer's recommendation)
Boiling water	6 ounces (170.1 grams)
Glitter	1 teaspoon (4.9 milliliters; or as desired)

1. Mix all the dry ingredients together.

2. Add fragrance oil and coloring to the boiling water.

3. Stir into the dry ingredients. When a paste forms, knead the dough for a few minutes. Add the glitter, and work into dough.

4. Form into little balls and flatten them to look like rocks, or roll out the dough and cut out shapes with cookie cutter.

5. Let dough dry. The dough rocks will dry very hard and give off fragrance for a month or two.

Lotion Bars

Home-crafters have been making these lotion bars for years. We use deodorant tubes as the containers for the lotion bars. This recipe makes 10 ounces (283.5 grams), or enough to fill 10 (1-ounce; 28.4-gram) push-up deodorant tubes.

Shea butter	2 ounces (56.7 grams)
Cocoa butter	2 ounces (56.7 grams)
Beeswax	4 ounces (113.4 grams)
Oil (your choice)	2 ounces (56.7 grams)
Fragrance or essential oil	1 teaspoon (4.9 milliliters)

1. In a saucepan over low heat, melt the butters slowly. Just before the butters are completely melted, remove from heat and stir until they finish melting.

2. Melt the beeswax in the microwave. When melted, add to the melted butters. Add oil and fragrance.

3. Stir well and pour into sterile deodorant tubes. Let sit on the counter to cool for several hours. When cool, put the caps on, and they're ready to roll.

Un-Petroleum Jelly

Years ago I found this recipe on the Internet. It makes a nice jelly like Vaseline. Use in recipes in place of Vaseline or lanolin. You can also use this on baby's bum to protect from diaper rash. This recipe makes 4 ounces (113.4 grams).

Beeswax	2 ounces (56.7 grams)
Oil (your choice)	2 ounces (56.7 grams)
Preservative	(see manufacturer's recommendation)

1. Place a bowl on the scale, and push the tare button. Weigh the wax.

2. In a disposable microwavable container, melt the wax on low heat until it's completely melted.

3. While the wax is melting, put another bowl on the scale and push the tare button. Weigh the oil.

4. When the wax has completely melted, pour the oil and preservative into the melted wax and stir well.

5. Pour mixture into a sterile jar and let sit on the counter overnight to cool. When completely cooled, place the cap on the jar, and it's ready to use.

> **PRETTY POINTER**
>
> Make the Un-Petroleum Jelly a diaper rash ointment by adding 1 teaspoon (4.9 milliliters) grapefruit essential oil. Do not use on babies under the age of 3 months, though.

Shower Sinus Tabs

These sinus tabs are perfect for those who suffer from allergies and head colds. Just throw a tab in the bottom of your tub where the water will hit it. While you take your shower, the vapors will help clear out your stuffed nose. You make them just like regular bath bombs, except you boil the water and use it to melt the menthol crystals. This recipe makes 24 (1-ounce; 28.4-gram) sinus tabs.

Baking soda	1 cup (236.6 milliliters)
Cornstarch	1 cup (236.6 milliliters)
Distilled water	¾ teaspoon (3.7 milliliters)
Menthol crystals	1 teaspoon (4.9 milliliters)
Sweet almond oil	1 ounce (28.4 grams)
Eucalyptus essential oil	1 teaspoon (4.9 milliliters)
Citric acid	½ cup (118.3 milliliters)

1. Measure the baking soda and cornstarch, and put in a large bowl. Mix together well.

2. Measure the distilled water, and bring it to a boil. Add menthol crystals, and stir until dissolved. Add the sweet almond oil and eucalyptus essential oil, and stir well.

3. Drizzle the liquids into the dry ingredients, and whisk together. Switch to an electric hand mixer and continue mixing until the liquids are well disbursed throughout the mixture.

4. Add the citric acid, and mix well.

5. Preheat the oven to 170°F. Using a bomb tapper or a candy mold, mold your shower tabs, pack them tight, and place them on a cookie sheet. *Turn off the oven* and put the shower tabs in the oven, and close the door for 1 hour.

6. After the tabs have been in the oven for an hour, remove them and using a knife, remove the tabs from the cookie sheet. Let the tabs air-dry overnight. The next day, wrap the tabs in foil candy wrappers.

SAFETY FIRST

Don't overdo the menthol crystals. They may smell mild now, but when hot water or heat hits them, they put off *lots* of vapors. One time I decided to make my shower sinus tabs stronger and added 1 full tablespoon (14.8 milliliters). When I opened the oven door, the smell made me light-headed and I went down on my knees. We had to open the windows and doors to air out the house! That batch went straight into the trash.

Take Care of Your Hair

This book wouldn't be complete if we didn't include a few hair product recipes!

Easy Hair Conditioner

This is a quick but very nice hair conditioner recipe. It leaves your hair soft and easy to wet comb. This recipe makes 16 ounces (453.6 grams).

Distilled water	14.4 ounces (408.2 grams)
Meadowfoam seed oil	.5 ounce (14.2 grams)
Conditioning emulsifier or *BTMS*	.8 ounce (22.7 grams)
Fragrance or essential oil	.2 ounce (5.7 grams)
Preservative	(see manufacturer's recommendation)

Prepare as directed in the Thick and Luscious Body Butter recipe in Chapter 7.

BEAUTY BIT

BTMS is a great conditioning pellet that also emulsifies. It's really cool and easy to work with.

After the emulsion has cooled, you may want to add 3 percent each of silk amino acid and honeyquat for extra shine and conditioning.

Conditioning Spray for Dry Hair

There are times when we want to refresh our hair and give it a little extra shine. The essential oils used in this conditioning spray help dry and brittle hair. Just lightly spray your hair when it feels dry, or use it after you've shampooed and your hair is still wet. This recipe makes 1 ounce (28.4 grams).

Perfumer's alcohol	1 ounce (28.4 grams)
Basil essential oil	10 drops
Lavender essential oil	10 drops
Geranium essential oil	10 drops
Chamomile essential oil	10 drops

1. Blend all the ingredients together, and pour into a fine-mist spray bottle.

2. Spray on your dog when he or she needs a little freshening.

Conditioning Spray for Oily Hair

For oily hair, you use a different blend of essential oils. These help slow the scalp from producing so much oil. Just lightly spray it on your hair when it's wet. This recipe makes 1 ounce (28.4 grams).

Perfumer's alcohol	1 ounce (28.4 grams)
Bergamot essential oil	10 drops
Clary sage essential oil	10 drops
Eucalyptus essential oil	10 drops
Geranium essential oil	10 drops

1. Weigh your alcohol, and count the drops of essential oil.

2. Blend all the ingredients together, and pour into a fine-mist spray bottle.

For Special Skin Treatment

At some time or another, nearly everyone has a rash or overly dried-out skin. For those times, we offer several useful recipes you'll wonder how you ever got along without!

Cracked Heels and Hands Balm

Are your hands and heels very chapped? This balm helps you soothe and heal the skin. This recipe makes 2 (8-ounce; 226.8-gram) jars or 4 (4-ounce; 113.4-gram) jars.

Candelilla wax	1.9 ounces (53.9 grams)
Shea butter	3.5 ounces (99.2 grams)
Lanolin	7 ounces (198.4 grams)
Black cumin seed oil	1.9 ounces (53.9 grams)
Meadowfoam seed oil	1.3 ounces (36.9 grams)
Vitamin E	.3 ounce (8.5 grams)
Skin-safe fragrance or essential oil	.2 ounce (5.7 grams)
Preservative	(see manufacturer's recommendation)

1. Place a bowl on the scale, and push the tare button. Weigh the wax and butter.

2. Place them in a microwavable bowl, and melt on low heat using short spurts. Just before the butter has completely melted, add lanolin and stir until they finish melting.

3. Put another bowl on the scale, and push the tare button. Weigh the oils, and add each one to the butter and wax mixture.

4. Add the vitamin E and stir well.

5. Let cool down to 110°F and add the fragrance and preservative. Pour into sterile jars.

6. To use, just before bed, coat hands and/or feet with balm and cover with socks or gloves overnight.

Rash Spray

Rashes are uncomfortable to say the least, and this spray will help soothe the irritated skin while it helps heal. This recipe makes 4 ounces (113.4 grams).

Fractionated coconut oil	4 ounces (113.4 grams)
Lavender essential oil	40 drops
Chamomile essential oil	40 drops
Geranium essential oil	40 drops

1. Place a cup or bowl on the scale, and push the tare button. Weigh the fraction-ated coconut oil and add the drops of essential oils. Pour into a fine-mist spray bottle.

2. Spray as needed on rashes.

Red Skin Balancing Spray

This spray helps return red skin blotches to normal. This recipe makes 4 ounces (113.4 grams).

Algae extract	1.8 ounces (51 grams)
Borage oil	.6 ounce (17 grams)
Evening primrose oil	.3 ounce (8.5 grams)
Jojoba oil	1.3 ounce (36.9 grams)

1. Place a bowl on the scale, and push the tare button. Weigh each ingredient one at a time, and pour them into a sterilized 4-ounce (113.4-gram) fine-mist sprayer bottle.

2. Spray on as needed.

Antifungal Cream

This lotion not only stops fungus growth, it also stops feet or underarms from smelling. This recipe makes 16 ounces (453.6 grams).

Aloe vera juice	6 ounces (170.1 grams)
Glycerin	.2 ounce (5.7 grams)
Coconut oil	3.5 ounces (99.2 grams)
Emu oil	1.1 ounces (31.2 grams)
Karanja oil	1.1 ounces (31.2 grams)
Neem oil	.6 ounce (17 grams)
Black cumin seed oil	1.6 ounces (45.4 grams)
Stearic acid	.5 ounce (14.2 grams)
Emulsifying wax	1.3 ounces (36.9 grams)
Rosemary oleo resin	1 teaspoon (4.9 milliliters)
Vitamin E	1 tablespoon (14.8 milliliters)
Neem extract	1 tablespoon (14.8 milliliters)
Essential oil blend	.3 ounce (8.5 grams)
Preservative	(see manufacturer's recommendation)

Essential oil blend:

Lavender essential oil	3.6 grams
Peppermint essential oil	2.4 grams
Ginger essential oil	2.5 grams

Prepare as directed in the Thick and Luscious Body Butter recipe in Chapter 7.

Arnica Balm

Have a backache, knee ache, or any kind of body ache? Try this balm. You'll be amazed at how quickly it relieves your aches and pains. Just rub the balm into the achy part, and go about your business. After a few minutes, you'll realize you're not hurting anymore, or not hurting as bad. The relief lasts up to 2 hours per application. I use this right before I mop my floors to avoid the resulting aches. This recipe makes 8 ounces (226.8 grams).

Triple-strength arnica-infused sunflower oil	7 ounces (198.4 grams)
Candelilla wax	.8 ounce (22.7 grams)
Essential oil pain blend	.25 ounce (7.1 grams)
Preservative	(see manufacturer's recommendation)

Essential oil blend:

Lavender essential oil	2.1 grams
Chamomile essential oil	.7 gram
Peppermint essential oil	2.2 grams
Ginger essential oil	.7 gram
Lemongrass essential oil	.7 gram
Helichrysum essential oil	.7 gram

1. Weigh the wax and add it to a saucepan. Set it over low heat and melt.

2. Weigh and add the oil to the melted wax. Let mixture cool down to 110°F, and add the preservative and essential oil blend. Pour into sterile jars.

3. The mixture will thicken as it cools. Place the caps on the jars nice and tight.

IN THE MIRROR

What makes this an essential oil pain blend? The lavender essential oil is used for numbing; the chamomile is anti-inflammatory; the peppermint adds heat; and the ginger, lemongrass, and helichrysum help nerve endings.

All-Purpose Hand Cream

This recipe may seem like it has some unusual ingredients, and in a way it does. Still, it's very healing and conditioning for the hands and elbows. This recipe makes 16 ounces (453.6 grams).

Aloe vera juice	6.4 ounces (181.4 grams)
Black cumin oil	1.6 ounces (45.4 grams)
Castor oil	.5 ounce (14.2 grams)
Yarrow-infused sunflower oil	1.6 ounces (45.4 grams)
Meadowfoam seed oil	1.6 ounces (45.4 grams)
Karanja oil	1.4 ounces (39.7 grams)
Neem oil	1.4 ounces (39.7 grams)
Stearic acid	.5 ounce (14.2 grams)
Emulsifying wax	.8 ounce (22.7 grams)
Rosemary oleo resin	.08 ounce (2.3 grams)
Vitamin E	.25 ounce (7.1 grams)
Essential oil	.2 ounce (5.7 grams)
Preservative	(see manufacturer's recommendation)

Prepare as directed in the Thick and Luscious Body Butter recipe in Chapter 7.

Rashes-and-More Cream

My grandson loved this cream when he wore diapers. He had very sensitive skin, and many of the creams and diaper-rash products burned and stung his skin. We would use this on him, and it didn't burn or irritate his delicate skin. This cream works on all types of rashes, helping soothe and heal irritated skin. This recipe makes 16 ounces (453.6 grams).

Aloe vera juice	12 ounces (340.2 grams)
Emu or ostrich oil	1.6 ounces (45.4 grams)
Emulsifying wax	.8 ounce (22.7 grams)
Stearic acid	.5 ounce (14.2 grams)
Z-Cote zinc oxide	1.1 ounces (31.2 grams)
Essential oil blend	.2 ounce (5.7 grams)
Preservative	(see manufacturer's recommendation)

Essential oil blend:

Lavender essential oil	.2 gram
German chamomile essential oil	.8 gram
Geranium essential oil	.8 gram
Carrot seed oil	2.7 grams
Bergamot essential oil	1.1 grams

Prepare as directed in the Thick and Luscious Body Butter recipe in Chapter 7.

Total Body Balm

Head-to-toe softness! This recipe makes 24 ounces (680.4 grams).

Cocoa butter	5.8 ounces (164.4 grams)
Shea butter	2.9 ounces (82.2 grams)
Candelilla wax	3.6 ounces (102.1 grams)
Fractionated coconut oil	5.8 ounces (164.4 grams)
Avocado oil	2.2 ounces (62.4 grams)
Emu oil	2.2 ounces (62.4 grams)
Jojoba oil	1.4 ounces (39.7 grams)
Vitamin E	.25 ounce (7.1 grams)
Fragrance or essential oil	.25 ounce (7.1 grams)
Preservative	(see manufacturer's recommendation)

Prepare as directed in the Dry Skin Facial Balm recipe in Chapter 6.

PRETTY POINTER

If you'd rather not use an animal product—emu oil—you can substitute meadowfoam seed oil instead.

Soothing Oils for Mature Skin

As we get older, our skin needs more help retaining oil to maintain soft skin. In this section, we give you a few intense oils that help mature skin stay soft and well moisturized all day long.

Velvet Skin Oil for Mature Skin

Rosehip seed oil is known to lighten the age and brown spots we all tend to get as we grow older. This oil is an excellent choice as an ingredient in facial soaps for mature skin. This recipe makes 4 ounces (113.4 grams).

Rosehip seed oil	1.2 ounces (34 grams)
Meadowfoam seed oil	.8 ounce (22.7 grams)
Peach kernel oil	.6 ounce (17 grams)
Macadamia nut oil	.6 ounce (17 grams)
Vitamin E	.8 ounce (22.7 grams)
Rosemary oleo resin	¼ teaspoon (1.2 milliliters)

Blend ingredients together and pour into a sterile bottle.

Nourishing Oil for Mature Skin

The oils in this recipe do a double duty because they add much-needed vitamins and nutriments. This recipe makes 4 ounces (113.4 grams).

Vitamin E	.4 ounce (11.3 grams)
Peach kernel oil	1.2 ounces (34 grams)
Rosehip seed oil	1 ounce (28.4 grams)
Macadamia nut oil	1 ounce (28.4 grams)
Evening primrose oil	1 ounce (28.4 grams)
Rosemary oleo resin	⅛ teaspoon (.6 milliliter)

Blend ingredients together and pour into a sterile bottle.

Scar Tissue Oil

We all have scars from surgeries or childhood injuries, perhaps. The recipes in this section help fade and minimize those scars. Once you've made the recipe, pour it into a small brown glass bottle, and keep bottle out of direct sunlight. (This helps it last longer.) Then simply apply twice a day to scars.

In addition to the Stretch Mark Oil recipe earlier in the chapter, these oils work on stretch marks, too.

Scar Tissue Oil

This oil helps to fade and diminish scars and smooth out the scar tissue. This recipe makes 2 ounces (56.7 grams).

Borage oil	.4 ounce (11.3 grams)
Thistle-infused safflower oil	.6 ounce (17 grams)
Vitamin E oil	1 ounce (28.4 grams)
Rosehip seed oil	.5 ounce (14.2 grams)
Vitamin A	.04 ounce (1.1 grams)

1. Blend ingredients together and pour into a sterile bottle.

2. Apply to scars twice a day.

Rosehip Scar Tissue Oil

This scar tissue oil offers a different blend of ingredients. It does wonders on scar tissue. This recipe makes 2 ounces (56.7 grams).

Thistle extract	.3 ounce (8.5 grams)
Black cumin seed oil	.2 ounce (5.7 grams)
Borage oil	.2 ounce (5.7 grams)
Vitamin E	1 ounce (28.4 grams)
Rosehip seed oil	.3 ounce (8.5 grams)
Vitamin A	.04 ounce (1.1 grams)

1. Blend ingredients together and pour into a sterile bottle.

2. Apply to scars twice a day.

Making an Essential Oil Blend

Many essential oils can work together to give you a desired effect. Zonella experimented with different amounts and different combinations until she found just the right blend. Here she shares the pain blend and the antifungal blend in larger amounts so you can use these blends in more of your formulas. She has used these blends for years in many of her products, and they do work!

Start with a sterile 8-ounce (226.8-gram) brown glass bottle. An 8-ounce bottle only holds about 7 ounces (198.4 grams) essential oil.

> **SAFETY FIRST**
>
> All essential oils need to be kept out of the light and out of plastic bottles. The plastic will break down as well as absorb into the essential oils. Always use brown glass bottles for your essential oils. If you order your essential oils and they come packaged in plastic, transfer them to brown glass bottles as soon as possible.

Essential Oil Blend for Pain Relief

This is Zonella's blend of essential oils she uses in her pain creams. This recipe makes 7 ounces (198.4 grams).

Lavender essential oil	2 ounces (56.7 grams)
Peppermint essential oil	2 ounces (56.7 grams)
Chamomile essential oil	.8 ounce (22.7 grams)
Lemongrass essential oil	.7 ounce (19.8 grams)
Ginger essential oil	.7 ounce (19.8 grams)
Helichrysum essential oil	.7 ounce (19.8 grams)

1. Blend the oils together and pour into a sterile bottle.

2. Store in a cool, dark place. To use, just weigh the amount you need.

> **PRETTY POINTER**
>
> Helichrysum essential oil is very expensive these days, so you might want to omit this essential oil from blends until the price comes back down. It's a wonderful and beneficial essential oil, but the price today makes it not cost-effective. You can buy a type of helichrysum essential oil from Liberty Naturals called *helichrysum gymnocephalum* for much less. It works just as well as the expensive type.

Antifungal Essential Oil Blend

This is Zonella's essential oil blend she uses for several of her formulations for fungus and body odor control. This recipe makes 7 ounces (198.4 grams).

Lavender essential oil	3 ounces (85 grams)
Peppermint essential oil	2 ounces (56.7 grams)
Ginger essential oil	2 ounces (56.7 grams)

1. Blend the oils together and pour into a sterile bottle.

2. Store in a cool, dark place. To use, just weigh the amount you need.

The Least You Need to Know

- For just about whatever beauty product you're looking for, you can find it in this book—or in this catch-all chapter of fun recipes!
- There are many fun projects for preteens and teens that you can share with them.
- Don't forget what you learned in the other chapters about sterilizing your containers, equipment, and workspace. That all applies here, too!

Glossary

allantoin   A substance that is very soothing on the skin.

aloe vera   The juice or gel, comes from the leaves of the aloe vera plant. It is a clear liquid that soothes and heals our skin. It is often used in cosmetics and after-sun care products.

alpha hydroxy acid   It comes from the natural sugars in fruits and milk. It is used to rejuvenate the skin.

amino acid   There are many types of amino acids. They come from proteins and many are essential for a healthy body.

analgesic   Pain relieving; a substance that relieves pain.

anhydrous   A liquid, such as an oil, or a formulation that does not contain water.

anti-inflammatory   Stops inflammation of the skin.

anti-irritant   Does not cause irritation of the skin or stops irritation.

antibacterial   Kills bacteria and can be used to treat infections.

antifungal   Stops the growth of fungi or mold.

antioxidant   A synthetic or natural material that slows oils becoming rancid and also slows the aging of skin cells.

antiperspirant   Stops the body from releasing sweat.

antiseptic   Prevents infections.

antispasmodic   Relieves muscle cramps.

antiviral   Does not allow a virus to grow.

aromatherapy   The use of essential oils to help with a person's emotions.

aromatic   Having a strong fragrance or odor.

ascorbic acid   Vitamin C in powder form.

astringent   A liquid used to tighten the skin and remove oils. An astringent is stronger than a toner.

beeswax   Wax obtained from the honeycomb. Used in candles, and to thicken lip balms and lipsticks.

bentonite clay   A white clay used in facial masks to absorb the excess oils.

bleaching   The part of the refining process that removes the color of an oil or fat. Red palm oil is bleached to take the red out of it.

botanical   Describes something related to a plant.

calendula (a.k.a. marigold)   An herb often used in fresheners, soothing creams, and sensitive skin products. Sometimes it is used in deodorants.

candelilla wax   A wax used to thicken balms and lipsticks. The wax on the market today doesn't actually come from the candelilla plant like you would expect, but it actually comes from the stems of a different plant in the same family called *Euphorbia Antisyphillitica*.

carnauba wax   A wax that comes from the fan palm and is used to thicken balms and lipsticks. It is harder than candelilla wax.

carrier oil   An oil that will penetrate the skin and is used to dilute and carry an essential oil or essential oil blend into the skin's tissues. Also used for infusing herbs.

carrot oil   A gold-colored oil that comes from the root of the carrot, not the seed.

carrot seed oil   An oil made from the seeds of carrots. It has many benefits for the hair and is used in lots of hair care products.

castor oil   An oil that comes from the castor bean. It's used in many cosmetics and soaps.

cetearyl alcohol   This is made from palm oil and is used in creams and lotions to add moisture to the skin.

chamomile   An herb used in many products for blond hair to enhance color and in cosmetics for inflamed and tender skin. It is also an antioxidant.

chandler   A person who makes and sells candles.

cicatrisant   A substance that helps to heal scar tissue.

citric acid   A natural powder ingredient that comes from citrus and pineapples. It lowers the pH levels in skin care products and also adds the fizz in bath bombs.

cleansing cream (a.k.a. cold cream)   A cream made for dissolving and removing makeup; it is applied to the face and then wiped off.

coffee grinder   An electric device that grinds coffee beans for making coffee. In our case we use this tool to grind oxides, micas, and powders together to make mineral makeup. It can also be use to grind dried herbs.

cold pressed   The process in which oils are extracted by machines. The process keeps the temperature below 125°F.

collagen   Proteins that keep our skin from sagging and wrinkling.

comedogenic   An oil that clogs pores. A noncomedogenic won't clog the pores.

conditioner   A creamy, moisturizing product to put on hair after shampooing to make it easier to detangle and comb

copra   It is the dried meat of a coconut. Coconut oil is obtained from the copra.

cosmetic   Products that we use on our bodies to cleanse or to enhance our appearance.

cosmetic grade   Ingredients that are FDA-approved for use in cosmetics.

cream   A formulation for our skin that is thicker than a lotion. A cream has more oils in it than a lotion.

cream rinse   A hair rinse used after shampooing that helps to detangle the hair.

cucumber   A vegetable often used in facial creams, lotions, and cleansers. Cucumbers have astringent and soothing properties.

D&C   Prefix showing that the FDA has approved a color for drug and cosmetic use.

deodorize   The process in which odors are removed.

dimethicone   A silicone that is an organic polymer that is a moisturizing emollient and used in skin and hair products.

elder flower   A flowering plant used in eye and skin creams for its astringent properties.

emollient   A substance that is soothing and softening to the skin and also protects the skin.

emulsifying wax   A wax used to combine oils with water when manufacturing lotions and creams.

emulsion   A mixture of oil and water that has been blended by using an emulsifying wax.

epidermis   The top outer layer of the skin.

Epsom salt   Magnesium sulfate. This draws toxins out of the body.

essential oil   An oil that's steamed or pressed from plant leaves, buds, or stems. These natural oils offer many benefits.

ewax   *See* emulsifying wax.

exfoliant   A product that gently removes dead skin cells.

expeller pressed   The extraction of oil using a machine to press the oil from a plant or seed. The heat never gets higher than 220°F.

FD&C   Prefix showing that a product has been approved to be used in Foods, Drugs, and Cosmetics.

fixative   A substance used to hold fragrance and essential oil, whose scent tends to fade, in a product such as soap, lotions, or candles.

fixed oils   Vegetable oils in their natural state. Olive oil, coconut oil, and sunflower oil, to name a few, are all fixed oils.

flash point   The temperature that heated essential or fragrance oil vapors will ignite when exposed to an open flame at a certain temperature. Example: A fragrance rated 200FP means it will not ignite when used in a candle, unless the temperature of the wax or container gets over 200°F.

floral water   *See* hydrosol.

formula   A recipe for cosmetics; usually shown in percentages.

fragrance oil   A synthetic oil that is made with aroma powders and essential oils in a synthetic base oil.

French talc   A white, silky-feeling, fine powder that is used as a filler in cosmetics. Helps other powders adhere to the skin.

glycerin   A by-product of soap.

grapefruit seed extract (GSE)   A liquid extracted from grapefruit seeds and used in some cosmetics as a preservative.

herb   Any plant or part of a plant used as a medicine, seasoning, or flavoring.

humectant   Describes something that absorbs water.

hydrolat   *See* hydrosol.

hydrosol   Also called floral water. This is the water left behind after the steam distilling of essential oils.

immersion blender   A long, skinny, handheld tool used to blend ingredients together.

INCI   International Nomenclature of Cosmetic Ingredients. The INCI name is required when labeling cosmetics marketed in the United States.

infusion   Steeping botanicals in oil or water.

insoluble   Describes something that will not dissolve in a liquid, such as water or alcohol.

Joy Wax   A wax blend of soy and other botanical waxes. Includes a very small percent of food grade paraffin wax. This wax is a name brand and only sold at Nature's Garden, an online business.

lanolin   A yellow sticky wax-type substance produced and secreted by sheep to protect their skin and wool. It is very conditioning to the skin.

lip balm   A thick substance applied to lips to soothe and moisturize.

magnesium stearate   A white, flat powder made from palm oil and magnesium salts. Used in filler bases for cosmetics.

melting point   The temperature at which a solid becomes a liquid.

micas   Once mined from the earth, these mineral powders are now made in labs under sterile conditions. Shiny and sparkly, they come in all colors.

mineral color corrector   A primer made from oxides and powders to correct skin tones or discolored blotches.

mineral color grind   A blend of micas and/or oxides to create a certain color.

mineral concealer   A cosmetic that covers under-eye darkness or blemishes.

mineral eye shadow   An eyelid colorant made of micas and oxides.

mineral eyeliner   Eyeliner made with oxides and micas as colorant for lining under eyes and on top of the eyelid.

mineral foundation   A blend of oxides and powders used to even facial skin tones.

mineral lip liner   Lip liner made with a blend of oxides and micas as a colorant for lining the lips.

mineral lipstick   Lipstick colored with a blend of oxides and micas, used to color lips.

mineral makeup   Makeup made of oxides, micas, and powders.

muscovado   A type of unrefined brown sugar. It has a strong molasses flavor.

oxides   Once mined from the earth, these minerals are now made in labs under sterile conditions. Oxides are flat (not sparkly), colored powders.

palm kernel stearin   A waxy hard oil that comes from the palm kernel.

panthenol   Vitamin B$_5$, good for hair and skin.

paraffin   A petroleum-based solid wax, used in candles and cosmetics.

peptide   A peptide is made up of two amino acids and is added to cosmetics to treat wrinkles.

pipette   A disposable plastic dropper used to add measured amounts to formulas.

refine   The process of removing impurities from natural, or crude, oils and butters.

retinol   Retinol is an acid made from vitamin A. It is an antioxidant and very important for our vision and growth of our bones.

rice powder   A natural light, white powder made from rice often used in mineral makeup as part of the base filler.

roller-ball bottles   Small glass bottles (usually $\frac{1}{3}$-ounce) with a roller ball on the top so you can roll a product onto your skin.

rose talc   Very similar to French talc. Also used as a filler for cosmetics.

rosemary oleoresin extract (ROE)   This is an extract, from the rosemary plant, used to extend the shelf life of oils and cosmetics.

sea salt   Salt produced by evaporation of seawater.

sebum   Oil produced by the body to keep skin moisturized. The lack of sebum produces dry skin.

sericite mica   A fine-grain, off-white mica that has a little sheen.

serum   A concentrated solution that is used on the face after cleansing.

silk mica   A very soft and silky-feeling white powder made from inorganic pigment powders.

sodium carbonate   Washing soda.

soy wax   A natural wax that comes from soybeans.

steam distillation   A process in which essential oils are extracted from plant materials using steam and pressure.

stearic acid   Obtained from animal and vegetable fats. Used for hardening or adding stiffness to soaps, candles, and lotions.

synthetic   Something that's artificially produced.

talc   Used as a powder to absorb oil and take the shine off skin.

tocopherol   Natural vitamin E. *See also* tocopheryl.

tocopheryl   Synthetic vitamin E. *See also* tocopherol.

toner   Gentler and not as drying as an astringent. Used after a cleanser to normalize the pH levels of skin.

tubes, push-up   1-ounce (28.4-gram) to 1.75-ounce (49.6-gram) tubes used for lotion bars and other hardened products like deodorant that push up from the bottom of the tube.

tubes, twist-up   1-ounce (28.4-gram) to 1.75-ounce (49.6-gram) tubes used for lotion bars and other hardened products like deodorant that twist up from the bottom of the tube.

turbinado sugar   Unrefined raw cane sugar that has been steam-cleaned. It is often used in sugar scrubs and body polishes.

turkey red oil (TRO)   Sulfonated castor oil. This oil is often used in bath oils because it disperses in water and does not leave a slick feel or a ring in the tub.

unflavored gelatin   A powder made mostly of proteins that is used in cooking for making a stable jelly.

unrefined   In a natural or original state.

vitamin C   *See* ascorbic acid.

water soluble   Dissolvable in water.

wildcrafted   Refers to herbs and botanicals grown in the wild without the use of pesticides or other chemicals.

xanthan gum   A natural carbohydrate gum used as a thickener.

zinc oxide   Soothes and heals the skin and is used in sun protection.

INCI Labeling Names

When making labels for your natural beauty products, you need to use the proper name, as dictated by the International Nomenclature of Cosmetic Ingredients (INCI). It includes the common name and then the botanical name.

The ingredients have to be arranged on the label in the order they're used. The ingredient at the top, used at a greater quantity, is followed by less-common ingredients, all the way down to the last ingredient, which is the least amount used. Any ingredient used in a quantity less than 1 percent does not need to be listed.

For an example, let's look at an herbal salve that contains the following ingredients:

Lanolin

Castor oil

Rice bran oil infused with calendula

Rice bran oil infused with chamomile

Rice bran oil infused with comfrey

Rice bran oil infused with neem leaf

Rice bran oil infused with black walnut hull

Wax

Shea butter

Emu oil

Hemp seed oil

Tamanu oil

The label will read:

>Ingredients: Lanolin, Castor (*Ricinus Communis*) Seed Oil, Rice (*Oryza Sativa*) Bran Oil (and) Calendula (*Calendula Officinalis*) Flower Extract, Rice (*Oryza Sativa*) Bran Oil (and) Chamomile (*Anthemis Nobilis*) Extract, Rice (*Oryza Sativa*) Oil (and) Comfrey (*Symphytum Officinalis*) Extract, Rice (*Oryza Sativa*) Oil (and) Neem (*Azadirachta Indica*) Leaf Extract, Rice (*Oryza Sativa*) Bran Oil (and) Black Walnut (*Juglans Nigra*) Shell Extract, Candelilla (*Euphorbia Cerifera*) Wax, Shea (*Butyrospermum Parkii*) Butter, Emu Oil, Hemp Seed (*Cannabis Sativa*) Oil, Tamanu (*Calophyllum Inophyllum*) Oil

The Ingredient and Its INCI Name

Acacia Concinna Extract

Acacia Dealbata Extract

Acerola (*Malpighia Glabra*) Extract

Acerola (*Malpighia Punicifolia*)

Agrimony (*Agrimonia Eupatoria*) Extract Alcohol, Denatured Alcohol, Perfumer's (SD Alcohol 40B)

Alfalfa (*Medicago Sativa*) Extract

Alfalfa (*Medicago Sativa*) Leaf Powder

Alkanet (*Alkanna Tinctoria*) Root Extract

Allantoin

Allspice (*Pimento Officinalis*) Oil

Almond, Sweet (Hydrogenated *Prunus Amygdalus Dulcis*) Butter

Almond, Sweet (*Prunus Amygdalus Dulcis*) Meal

Almond, Sweet (*Prunus Amygdalus Dulcis*) Oil

Aloe (*Cocos Nucifera* [Coconut] Oil and *Barbadensis* Leaf Extract) Butter

Aloe Vera (*Barbadensis*) Extract

Aloe Vera (*Barbadensis*) Leaf Juice

Aloe Vera (*Barbadensis*) Leaf Powder

Aloe Vera Gel—varies; check manufacturer for exact ingredients

American Centaury (*Sabbatia Angularis*) Extract

Amla (*Emblica Officinalis*) Powder

Amla (*Emblica Officinalis*) Oil

Amyris (*Amyris Balsamifera*) Oil

Angelica (*Angelica Archangelica*) Oil

Anhydrous Lanolin (Lanolin)

Anise (*Pimpinella Anisum*) Extract

Anise (*Pimpinella Anisum*) Fruit Oil

Annatto Powder (*Bixa Orellana*)

Annona Muricata Extract

Anthyllis Vulneraria Extract

Antioxidant (Vitamin E; ROE; and T-50)

Antique Copper Mica

Antique Silver Mica

Apple (*Pyrus Malus*) Extract

Apple (*Pyrus Malus*) Peel Wax

Apple (*Pyrus Malus*) Water

Apple Cider Vinegar (Acetic Acid)

Apricot (*Prunus Armeniaca*) Kernel Oil

Apricot (*Prunus Armeniaca*) Seed Powder

Aqua (Water)

Argan (*Argania Spinosa*) Oil

Arnica (INCI of oil arnica is infused in [and] *Arnica Montana* Flower Extract)

Arrowroot (*Maranta Arundinacea*) Extract

Arrowroot (*Maranta Arundinacea*) Powder

Ascorbic Acid

Atlas Cedarwood (*Cedrus Atlantica*) Bark Oil

Avocado (Hydrogenated *Persea Gratissima*) Butter

Avocado (*Persea Gratissima*) Butter

Avocado (*Persea Gratissima*) Oil

Avocado (*Persea Gratissima*) Purée

Awhh Purple (Mica [and] Iron Oxide [and] Titanium Dioxide [and] Glycerin)

Aztec Marigold (*Tagetes Erecta*) Extract

Babassu (*Orbignya Oleifera*) Seed Oil

Baby Blue (Iron Oxide [and] Titanium Dioxide [and] Glycerin)

Baby Pink (Mica [and] Titanium Dioxide [and] Glycerin)

Baby Roses (Iron Oxide, Titanium Dioxide [and] Glycerin)

Baking Soda (*Sodium Bicarbonate*) Powder

Balm Mint (*Melissa Officinalis*) Distillate

Balm Mint (*Melissa Officinalis*) Extract

Balm Mint (*Melissa Officinalis*) Oil

Balm of Gilead (*Commiphora Gileadensis*) Extract

Balsam, Bulgaria (*Pinus Balsamea*) Oil

Balsam, Canada (*Abies Balsamea*)

Balsam, Copaiba (*Copaifera Officinale*) Root Powder

Balsam of Peru (*Myroxylon Pereirae*) Resin

Baobab (*Adansonia Digitata*) Oil

Barley (*Hordeum Vulgare*) Leaf Juice

Barley (*Hordeum Vulgare*) Root Extract

Basil (*Ocimum Basilicum*) Extract

Basil (*Ocimum Basilicum*) Oil

Basil, Holy (*Ocimum Sanctum*) Oil

Basswood (*Tilia Americana*) Extract

Bay (*Pimenta Racemosa*) Oil

Bayberry (*Myrica Cerifera*) Extract

Bayberry (*Myrica Cerifera*) Leaf Extract

Bayberry (*Myrica Cerifera*) Wax

Bearberry (*Arctostaphylos Uva Ursi*) Extract

Bee Balm (*Monarda Didyma*) Extract

Bee Balm (*Monarda Didyma*) Oil

Beef Tallow

Beeswax, white pastilies (*Cera Alba*)

Beet (*Beta Vulgaris*) Root Powder

Bentonite Clay

Benzaldehyde

Benzoin (*Styrax Benzoin*) Extract

Benzoin (*Styrax Benzoin*) Gum

Benzyl Benzoate USP

Bergamot (*Citrus Aurantium Bergamia*) Oil

Betula Platyphylla Japonica

Butylated Hydroxytoluene (BHT)

Bilberry (*Vaccinium Myrtillus*) Extract

Birch (*Betula Alba*) Bark Extract

Birch (*Betula Alba*) Leaf Extract

Birch (*Betula Alba*) Oil

Bitter Almond (*Prunus Amygdalus Amara*) Extract

Bitter Almond (*Prunus Amygdalus Amara*) Oil

Bitter Cherry (*Prunus Cerasus*) Extract

Bitter Cherry (*Prunus Cerasus*) Oil

Bitter Orange (*Citrus Aurantium Amara*) Extract

Bitter Orange (*Citrus Aurantium Amara*) Flower Distillate

Bitter Orange (*Citrus Aurantium Amara*) Flower Extract

Bitter Orange (*Citrus Aurantium Amara*) Oil

Bitter Orange (*Citrus Aurantium Amara*) Peel Extract

Black Cohosh (*Cimicifuga Racemosa*)

Black Cohosh (*Cimicifuga Racemosa*) Extract

Black Cumin (*Nigelia Sativa*) Seed Oil

Black Currant (*Ribes Nigrum*) Extract

Black Currant (*Ribes Nigrum*) Oil

Black Locust (*Robinia Pseudocacia*) Extract

Black Mustard (*Brassica Nigra*) Extract

Black Oxide (Iron Oxide)

Black Pepper (*Piper Nigrum*) Extract

Black Pepper (*Piper Nigrum*) Oil

Black Walnut (*Juglans Nigra*) Extract

Black Walnut (*Juglans Nigra*) Shell Extract

Blackberry (*Rubus Fruticosus*) Extract

Blackberry (*Rubus Fruticosus*) Leaf Extract

Blackberry (*Rubus Fruticosus*) Seeds

Bladderwrack (*Fucus Vesiculosus*) Powder

Blessed Thistle (*Carbenia Benedicta*) Extract

Blood Orange (*Citrus Aurantium Dulcis*) Oil

Blue Chamomile (*Chamomilla Recutita*) Flower Oil

Blue Cohosh (*Caulophyllum Thalictroides*)

Blue Flag (*Iris Versicolor*) Extract

Blue Sky Blue (Dioxide [and] Glycerin)

Borage (*Borago Officinalis*) Extract

Borage (*Borago Officinalis*) Seed Oil

Borax

Bourbon Vanilla (*Vanilla Planifolia*) Extract

Brahmi (*Bacopa Monniera*) Powder

Brazil (*Bertholletia Excelsa*) Nut Oil

Bright Gold (Mica)

Broom (*Cytisus Scoparius*) Extract

Brown Oxide (Iron Oxide)

Brown Sugar (Sucrose)

BTMS Emulsifier (Behentrimonium Methosulfate, Cetearyl Alcohol)

Buckbean (*Menyanthes Trifoliata*) Extract

Buckthorn (*Frangula Alnus*)

Buckthorn (*Frangula Alnus*) Extract

Buckwheat (*Polygonum Fagopyrum*) Extract

Bugloss (*Lycopsis Arvensis*) Extract

Bulgarian Lavender (*Lavandula Angustifolia*) Oil

Burdock (*Arctium Lappa*) Extract

Burdock (*Arctium Lappa*) Seed Oil

Burdock (*Arctium Majus*) Extract

Burdock (*Arctium Minus*) Extract

Butcherbroom (*Ruscus Aculeatus*) Extract

Buttermilk

Buttermilk Powder

Cabbage Rose (*Rosa Centifolia*) Extract

Cabbage Rose (*Rosa Centifolia*) Oil

Cabbage Rose (*Rosa Centifolia*) Water

Cactus (*Cereus Grandiflorus*) Extract

Cade (*Juniperus Oxycedrus* Wood) Oil

Cajeput (*Melaleuca Leucadendron*) Oil

Calamus (*Acorus Calamus*) Extract

Calamus (*Acorus Calamus*) Root Powder

Calcium Carbonate

Calendula (*Calendula Officinalis*) Flower Extract preceded with the INCI of oil used for the infusion

Calendula (*Calendula Officinalis*) Flower Petals

California Nutmeg (*Torreya Californica*) Extract

California Nutmeg (*Torreya Californica*) Oil

Camelina (*Camelina Sativa*) Seed Oil

Camellia (*Camellia Oleifera*) Extract

Camellia (*Camellia Japonica*) Oil

Camellia (*Camellia Kissii*) Oil

Camellia (*Camellia Sinensis*) Oil

Camphor (*Cinnamomum Camphora*) Bark Oil

Candelilla (*Euphorbia Cerifera*) Wax

Canola (*Brassica Campestris*) Oil—also known as rapeseed

Caraway (*Carum Carvi*) Extract

Caraway (*Carum Carvi*) Oil

Caraway (*Carum Carvi*) Seed Oil

Cardamom (*Elettaria Cardamomum*) Extract

Cardamon (*Elettaria Cardamomum*) Oil

Carnauba (*Copernicia Cerifera*) Wax

Carrageenan (*Chondrus Crispus*)

Carrot (*Daucus Carota Sativa*) Root Extract preceded by INCI of the oil the carrot is infused in

Carrot (*Daucus Carota Sativa*) Seed Oil

Cascara (*Rhamnus Purshiana*) Extract

Castor (*Ricinus Communis*) Seed Oil

Castor (*Sulfated Ricinus Communis*) Seed Oil—also known as Turkey Red

Catnip (*Nepeta Cataria*) Extract preceded with INCI of the oil the catnip is infused in

Catnip (*Nepeta Cataria*) Oil

Cedarleaf (*Thuja Occidentalis*) Oil

Cedarwood (*Juniperus Virginiana*) Oil

Celandine (*Chelidonium Majus*) Extract

Century (*Agave Americana*) Extract

Cetearyl Octanoate

Cetyl Alcohol NF

Cetyl Octanoate

Cetyl PPG-2 Isodeceth-7 Carboxylate

Chamomile (*Anthemis Nobilis*) Extract preceded with INCI of the oil used for infusion

Chamomile, German (*Matricaria Chamomilla*) Oil

Chamomile, German (*Matricaria Chamomilla*) Water

Chamomile, Maroc (*Ormenis Multicaulis*) Oil

Chamomile, Roman (*Anthemis Nobilis*) Oil

Chamomile, Roman (*Anthemis Nobilis*) Water

Chaparral (*Larrea Divaricata*) Extract

Chaparral (*Larrea Mexicana*) Extract

Cherry (*Prunus Avium*) Kernel Oil

Chestnut (*Castanea Sativa*) Extract

Chia (*Salvia Hispanica*) Oil

Chickweed (*Stellaria Media*) Extract

Chicory (*Cichorium Intybus*) Extract

Chicory (*Cichorium Intybus*) Leaf Extract

Chinese Angelica (*Angelica Polymorpha Sinensis*) Extract

Chinese Hibiscus (*Hibiscus Rosa-Sinensis*) Extract

Chinese Magnolia (*Magnolia Biondii*) Bark Extract

Chinese Magnolia (*Magnolia Biondii*) Extract

Chlorophyll

Chromium Oxide Green (Iron Oxide)

Cinnamon (*Cinnamomum Cassia*) Bark

Cinnamon (*Cinnamomum Cassia*) Extract

Cinnamon (*Cinnamomum Cassia*) Oil

Cinnamon (*Cinnamomum Zeylanicum*) Bark Powder

Cinnamon (*Cinnamomum Zeylanicum*) Leaf Oil

Citric Acid

Citronella (*Cymbopogon Nardus*) Oil

Citrus Junos Oil

Citrus Medica Limonium

Clary Sage (*Salvia Sclarea*) Extract

Clary Sage (*Salvia Sclarea*) Oil

Clay, Bentonite

Clay, Glacial (Canadian Colloidal Clay [and] Propylene Glycol, Diazolidinyl Urea, Iodopropynyl Butylcarbamate)

Clay, Red (Montmorillonite)

Clay, White (Kaolin)

Clematis Vitalba Extract

Clintonia Borealis Extract

Clove (*Eugenia Caryophyllus*) Bud Oil

Clove (*Eugenia Caryophyllus*) Leaf Oil

Clove (*Eugenia Caryophyllus*) Oil

Clover (*Trifolium Pratense*) Extract

Cocoa (*Theobroma Cacao*) Butter

Coconut (*Cocos Nucifera*) Cream

Coconut (*Cocos Nucifera*) Oil

Coconut (*Cocos Nucifera*) Purée

Coconut (*Cocos Nucifera*) Shell Powder

Coconut, Fractionated (Caprylic/Capric Triglyceride) Oil

Coffea Robusta Extract

Coffee (*Coffea Arabica* Seed Oil [and] Hydrogenated Vegetable Oil) Bean Butter

Colloidal Oatmeal (*Avena Sativa*) Kernel Flour

Colocynth (*Citrullus Colocynthis*)

Colocynth (*Citrullus Colocynthis*) Extract

Coltsfoot (*Tussilago Farfara*) Extract

Coltsfoot (*Tussilago Farfara*) Leaf Extract

Combretum Micranthum Extract

Comfrey (*Symphytum Officinale*) Extract

Comfrey (*Symphytum Officinale*) Leaf Extract

Comfrey (*Symphytum Officinale*) Leaf Powder

Comfrey (*Symphytum Officinale*) Root Powder

Coneflower (*Echinacea Angustifolia*) Extract

Coneflower (*Echinacea Angustifolia*) Leaf Extract

Coneflower (*Echinacea Pallida*) Extract

Coneflower (*Echinacea Purpurea*) Extract

Coneflower (*Echinacea Purpurea*) Root Extract

Copaiba Balsam (*Copaifera Officinalis*) Resin

Coriander (*Coriandrum Officinalis*) Oil

Coriander (*Coriandrum Sativum*) Extract

Coriander (*Coriandrum Sativum*) Oil

Coriander (*Coriandrum Sativum*) Seed Oil

Corn (*Zea Mays*) Cob Meal

Corn (*Zea Mays*) Flour

Corn (*Zea Mays*) Meal

Corn (*Zea Mays*) Oil

Corn (*Zea Mays*) Starch

Corn Poppy (*Papaver Rhoeas*) Extract

Cornflower (*Centaurea Cyanus*) Extract

Cornmint (*Mentha Arbensis*) Oil

Cornsilk Powder (*Zea Mays*)

Cottonseed (*Gossypium*) Oil

Couch Grass (*Agropyron Repens*) Extract

Coviox T-50 (*Tocopherol*) Oil

Cream (Bovine Butterfat)

Cucumber (*Cucumis Sativus*) Fruit

Cucumber (*Cucumis Sativus*) Juice

Cudweed (*Gnaphalium Polycephalum*) Extract

Cumin (*Cuminum Cyminum*) Extract

Curled Dock (*Rumex Crispus*) Extract

Currant (*Ribes Rubrum*) Extract

Cyclomethicone

Cyperus Rotundus Extract

Cypress (*Cupressus Sempervirens*) Nut Extract

Cypress (*Cupressus Sempervirens*) Oil

Cypress, Blue (*Callistris Intratropica*) Oil

Daffodil (*Narcissus Pseudo-Narcissus*) Extract

Daisy (*Bellis Perennis*) Extract

Damar (*Shorea Robusta*)

Dandelion (*Taraxacum Officinale*) Extract

Dandelion (*Taraxacum Officinale*) Root

Date (*Phoenix Dactylifera*) Extract

Dead Sea Clay (*Kaolinite*)

Dead Sea Salt (Sodium Chloride)

Denatured Alcohol

Dendritic (Sodium Chloride)

Dill Weed (*Peucedanum Graveolens*)

Dimethicone

Dipropylene Glycol USP

Dog Rose (*Rosa Canina*) Hips Extract

Dog Rose (*Rosa Canina*) Hips Oil

Dog Rose (*Rosa Canina*) Leaf Extract

Dog Rose (*Rosa Canina*) Seed Extract

DPG USP (Dipropylene Glycol)

Dry-Flo AF (Corn Starch Modified)

Dulcamara (*Solanum Dulcamara*) Extract

Eastern Pine (*Pinus Strobus*) Cone Extract

Eastern Pine (*Pinus Strobus*) Extract

Ecballium Elaterium Extract

EDTA, Tetrasodium

Elder Flower (*Sambucus Nigra*)

Elecampane (*Inula Helenium*) Extract

Elemi (*Canarium Luzxonicum*) Oil

Eleuthero Ginseng (*Acanthopanax Senticosus*) Extract

Elm (*Ulmus Campestris*) Extract

Emu Oil

Emulsifying Wax NF (Cetearyl Alcohol and Polysorbate 60)

English Oak (*Quercus Robur*) Extract

Epsom Salt USP (Magnesium Sulfate)

Eucalyptus (*Eucalyptus Citriodora*) Oil

Eucalyptus (*Eucalyptus Globulus*) Extract

Eucalyptus (*Eucalyptus Globulus*) Oil

European Ash (*Fraxinus Excelsior*) Extract

Evening Primrose (*Oenothera Biennis*) Extract

Evening Primrose (*Oenothera Biennis*) Oil

Everlasting (*Helichrysum Arenarium*) Extract

Everlasting (*Helichrysum Italicum*) Extract

Everlasting (*Helichrysum Stoechas*) Extract

Faba (*Vicia Faba*) Bean Extract

Fennel (*Foeniculum Vulgare*) Seed Powder

Fennel, Sweet (*Foeniculum Vulgare Dulce*) Oil

Fenugreek (*Trigonella Foenum-Graecum*) Extract

Feverfew (*Chrysanthemum Parthenium*) Extract

Fig (*Ficus Carica*) Extract

Figwort (*Scrophularia Nodosa*) Extract

Fir Needle (*Abies Sibirica*) Oil

Flavor Oils (all) (Flavor)

Flax Seed (*Linum Usitatissimum*) Seed Oil

Foraha Oil (Tamanu Oil)

Fractionated Coconut (Caprylic/Capric Triglyceride) Oil

Fractionated Shea (*Butyrospermum Parkii*) Oil

Fragrance Oils (all) (Fragrance)

Frankincense (*Olibanum*) Oil

Frankincense, India (*Boswellia Carteri*) Oil

Frankincense Oil 10% in Jojoba (*Simmondsia Chinensis* [Jojoba] Seed Oil [and] *Olibanum* [Frankincense] Oil)

French Rose (*Rosa Gallica*) Extract

Galbanum (*Ferula Galbaniflua*) Extract

Galbanum (*Ferula Galbaniflua*) Resin Oil

Galbanum Oil 10% in Jojoba (*Simmondsia Chinensis* [Jojoba] Seed Oil [and] *Ferula Galbaniflua* [Galbanum] Resin Oil)

Garden Balsam (*Impatiens Balsamina*) Extract

Garden Balsam (*Impatiens Balsamina*) Leaf Extract

Garlic (*Allium Sativum*) Oil

Geranium (*Pelargonium Graveolens*) Oil

Geranium Rose (*Pelargonium Graveolens Roseum*) Oil

Germall Plus (Diazolidinyl Urea, Iodopropynl Butylcarbamate)

Germall Plus, Liquid (Propylene Glycol, Diazolidinyl Urea, Iodopropynl Butylcarbamate) Liquid

German Blue Chamomile (*Matricaria Recutita*) Flower Water

German Blue Chamomile (*Matricaria Recutita*) Oil

Germander (*Teucrium Scorodonia*) Extract

Ginger (*Zingiber Officinale*) Extract

Ginger (*Zingiber Officinale*) Root Oil

Ginger (*Zingiber Officinale*) Root Powder

Ginseng, Panax (*Eleutherococcus Senticocus*)

Glacial Clay (Glacial Marine Clay)

Glycerin

Glyceryl Monostearate (Glyceryl Stearate)

Glycolic Acid 70% Solution (Glycolic Acid [and] Water)

Goat Butter

Goat Milk

Goatweed (*Aegopodium Podagraria*) Extract

Gold of Pleasure (*Camelina Sativa*) Oil

Goldenrod (*Solidago Odora*) Extract

Goldenrod (*Solidago Virgaurea*) Extract

Goldenseal (*Hydrastis Canadensis*) Extract

Goldenseal (*Hydrastis Canadensis*) Root Extract

Gotu Kola (*Centella Asiatica*)

Gourd (*Cucurbitaceae*) Extract

Grape (*Vitis Vinifera*) Fruit

Grape Seed (*Vitis Vinifera*) Oil

Grapefruit (*Citrus Grandis*) Oil

Grapefruit (*Citrus Grandis*) Peel

Grapefruit (*Citrus Grandis*) Seed Extract (GSE)

Green Clay, French (Montmorillonite)

Green Illite, Clay (Illite Clay)

Green Tea (*Camellia Sinensis*) Leaf

Green Tea Leaf Powder (*Camellia Sinensis*) Leaf Powder

GSE (Grapefruit Seed Extract)

Guar (*Cyanopsis Tetragonoloba*) Gum

Hazelnut (*Corylus Americana*) Oil

Hazelnut (*Corylus Avellana*) Oil

Heather (*Calluna Vulgaris*) Extract

Hedge Parsley (*Anthriscus Sylvestris*) Extract

Helianthus Tuberosus Extract

Helichrysum (*Helichrysum Gymnocephalum*) Oil

Helichrysum (*Helichrysum Italicum*) Flower Extract

Helichrysum (*Helichrysum Italicum*) Oil

Helichrysum (*Helichrysum Italicum*) Petals

Hemp Seed Butter (*Cannabis Sativa* Seed Oil [and] Hydrogenated Vegetable Oil)

Hemp Seed (*Cannabis Sativa*) Oil

Henna (*Lawsonia Inermis*) Extract

Herb Robert (*Geranium Robertianum*) Extract

Hibiscus (*Militaris*) Extract

Hibiscus (*Rosa Sinensis Linn*)

Hibiscus (*Sabdariffa*) Extract

Hibiscus (*Syriacus*) Extract

Holly (*Ilex Aquifolium*) Extract

Honey

Honey Powder (Fructose, Maltodextrin)

Honeysuckle (*Lonicera Caprifolium*) Extract

Honeysuckle (*Lonicera Japonica*) Extract

Honeysuckle (*Lonicera Japonica*) Leaf Extract

Hops (*Humulus Lupulus*)

Hops (*Humulus Lupulus*) Extract

Hops (*Humulus Lupulus*) Oil

Horehound (*Marrubium Vulgare*) Extract

Horse Chestnut (*Aesculus Hippocastanum*) Bark Extract

Horse Chestnut (*Aesculus Hippocastanum*) Extract

Horseradish (*Cochlearia Armoracia*) Extract

Horsetail (*Equisetum Arvense*) Extract

Horsetail (*Equisetum Arvense*) Leaf Extract

Horsetail (*Equisetum Hiemale*) Extract

Houseleek (*Sempervivum Tectorum*) Extract

Hunter Green (Iron Oxide [and] Glycerin)

Hyacinth (*Hyacinthus Orientalis*) Extract

Hybrid Safflower (*Carthamus Tinctorius*) Oil

Hybrid Sunflower (*Helianthus Annuus*) Oil

Hydrated Chromium Oxide Green (Iron Oxide [and] Glycerin)—this is a teal color

Hydrocotyl (*Centella Asiatica*) Extract

Hydrolyzed Oat Protein (Hydrolyzed Oat [*Avena Sativa*] [and] Glycerin [and] Phenoxyethanol [and] Water)

Hydrolyzed Silk

Hydrolyzed Wheat Protein (Hydroxypropyl Polysiloxane)

Hydrosol, Bulgarian (*Rosa Damascene* Distillate)

Hydrosol, Chamomile (*Chamaemelum Nobiel* Distillate)

Hydrosol, Cistus Labdanum (*Cistus Ladaniferus* [Rock Rose] Distillate)

Hydrosol, Lemon Balm (*Melissa Officinalis* [Lemon Balm] Distillate)

Hydrosol, Neroli (*Citrus Aurantium* [Neroli] Distillate)

Hydrosol, Rose Damascena (*Rose Damascena* [Rose] Distillate)

Hydrosol, Rosemary Verbenone (*Rosmarinus Officinalis* [Rosemary] Distillate)

Hydrosol, Witch Hazel (*Hamamelis Virginiana* [Witch Hazel] Distillate)

Hydrosol, Yarrow (*Achillea Millefolium* [Yarrow] Distillate)

Hydroxy Benzoxathiolone

Hyptis Suaveolens Oil

Hyssop (*Hyssopus Officinalis*) Extract

Hyssop (*Hyssopus Officinalis*) Oil

Iceland Moss (*Cetraria Islandica*) Extract

Illipe (*Shorea Stenoplera*) Seed Butter

Indian Cress (*Tropaeolum Majus*) Extract

Indian Hemp (*Apocynum Cannabinum*) Extract

Indigo Bush (*Dalea Spinosa*) Oil

Indigofera Tinctoria Extract

IPM (Isopropyl Myristate)

Isopropyl Myristiate

Ivy (*Hedera Helix*) Extract

Jaborandi (*Pilocarpus Pennatifolius*) Extract

Jalap (*Ipomoea Purga*) Resin

Jambul (*Eugenia Cumini*) Extract

Japanese Angelica (*Angelica Acutiloba*) Extract

Japanese Quince (*Chaenomeles Japonica*) Extract

Jasmine (*Jasminum Officinale*) Oil

Jasmine Absolute (*Jasminum Officinale*) Extract

Jojoba (Hydrogenated *Simmondsia Chinensis*) Beads

Jojoba (*Simmondsia Chinensis*) Oil

Juniper Berries (*Juniperus Communis*) Berries

Juniper Berry Oil (*Juniperus Communis* [Juniper]) Fruit Oil

Kaolin Clay (all) (Kaolinite)

Karanja Oil (*Pongamma Glabra* [Karanja] Oil)

Kelp, Atlantic (*Laminaria Digitata*) Powder

Kelp, Norwegian (*Ascophyllum Nososom*) Powder

Kiwi (*Actinidia Chinensis*) Fruit

Kiwi (*Actinidia Chinensis*) Seed Oil

Kiwi (*Actinidia Chinensis*) Water

Kokum (*Garcinia Indica*) Seed Butter

Kukui (*Aleurites Moluccana*) Nut Oil

Labdanum (*Cistus Labdaniferus*)

Labdanum (*Cistus Labdaniferus*) Oil

Labrador Tea (*Ledum Groenlandicum*) Extract

Labrador Tea (*Ledum Palustre*) Extract

Lactic Acid

Lady's Mantle (*Alchemilla Vulgaris*) Extract

Lady's Slipper (*Cypripedium Pubescens*) Extract

Lady's Thistle (*Silybum Marianum*) Extract

Lady's Thistle (*Silybum Marianum*) Fruit Extract

Lanolin

Lard

Laurel (*Laurus Nobilis*) Extract

Laurel (*Laurus Nobilis*) Oil

Lavandin (*Lavandula Hybrida*) Oil

Lavandin Grosso (*Lavandula Hybrida Grosso* [Lavender] Oil)

Lavender (*Lavandula Angustifolia*) Oil

Lavender (*Lavandula Angustifolia*) Water

Lavender Fields (Iron Oxide [and] Titanium Dioxide [and] Glycerin)

Lemon (*Citrus Medica Limonum*) Oil

Lemon (*Citrus Medica Limonum*) Peel Extract

Lemon Verbena (*Lippia Citriodora*) Extract

Lemongrass (*Cymbopogon Schoenanthus*) Oil

Lentil (*Lens Esculenta*) Extract

Lesquerella Fendleri Oil

Lettuce (*Lactuca Scariola Sativa*) Extract

Lettuce (*Lactuca Scariola Sativa*) Juice

Lichen (*Usnea Barbata*) Extract

Licorice (*Glycyrrhiza Glabra*)

Licorice (*Glycyrrhiza Glabra*) Extract

Lilac (*Syringa Vulgaris*) Extract

Lime (*Citrus Aurantifolia*) Oil

Lime (*Citrus Aurantifolia*) Peel Extract

Linden (*Tilia Cordata*) Extract

Linden (*Tilia Cordata*) Oil

Linden (*Tilia Cordata*) Water

Linden (*Tilia Cordata*) Wood Extract

Linden (*Tilia Platyphyllos*)

Linden (*Tilia Platyphyllos*) Extract

Linden (*Tilia Tomentosa*) Extract

Linden (*Tilia Vulgaris*) Extract

Linoleamidopropyl Dimethylamine Lactate

Linseed (*Linum Usitatissimum*) Oil

LiquaPar Optima (Phenoxyethanol, Methylparaben, Isobutylparaben, Butylparaben)

Liquid Germall (Propylene Glycol, Diazolidinyl Urea, Iodoprophynl Butycarbamate) Plus

Liquid Shea (*Butyrospermum Parkii*) Oil

Lithospermum Erythrorhizone Extract

Lithospermum Officinale Extract

Litsea Cubeba Fruit Oil

Locust Bean (*Ceratonia Siliqua*) Gum

Logwood (*Haematoxylon Campechianum*) Extract

Logwood (*Haematoxylin Campechianum*) Powder

Loquat (*Eriobotrya Japonica*) Extract

Loquat (*Eriobotrya Japonica*) Leaf Extract

Lotus Corniculatus Extract

Lovage (*Levisticum Officinale*) Extract

Lovage (*Levisticum Officinale*) Oil

Luffa Cylindrica Extract

Lungwort (*Pulmonaria Officinalis*) Extract

Lupin (*Lupinus Albus*) Extract

Lupin (*Lupinus Albus*) Oil

Lupin (*Lupinus Albus*) Oil Unsaponifiables

Lupin (*Lupinus Luteus*) Extract

Macadamia (*Macadamia Ternifolia*) Seed Oil

Magnesium Carbonate

Maiden Hair Fern (*Adiantum Capillus Veneris*) Extract

Mallow (*Malva Sylvestris*) Extract

Mallow (*Malva Sylvestris*) Leaf Powder

Mallow, Musk (*Malva Moschata*) Extract

Mandarin Orange (*Citrus Nobilis*) Peel Oil

Mango (*Mangifera Indica*) Seed Butter

Mango (*Mangifera Indica*) Seed Oil

Manihot Utilissima Extract

Manuka (*Leptospermum Scoparium*) Oil

Maritime Pine (*Pinus Pinaster*) Extract

Marshmallow (*Althea Officinalis*) Root Powder

Massoy (*Cryptocarya Massoy*) Bark Oil

Matricaria (*Chamomilla Recutita*) Extract

Matricaria (*Chamomilla Recutita*) Oil

May Chang (*Litsea Cubeba*) Oil

MEA-PPG-6-Laureth-6-Carboxylate

Meadowfoam (*Limnanthes Alba*) Seed Oil

Meadowsweet (*Spiraea Ulmaria*) Extract

Melaleuca Leucadendron Cajaputi (Cajeput)

Melissa; Lemon Balm (*Melissa Officinalis*) Oil

Menthol Crystals

Menthyicellulose

Methylsulfonyimethane (Dimethyl Sulfone)

Mica

Milk

Milk Powder (Whole Dry Milk)

Milk Powder, Skim (Nonfat Dry Milk)

Mineral (*Paraffinum Liquidum*) Oil

Mixed Tocopherols (Tocopherol)

Monoi de Tahiti (*Cocos Nucifera* [Coconut] Oil [and] *Gardenia Tahitensis* [Tiare] Flower Extract) Oil

MSM (Dimethyl Sulfone)

Mugwort (*Artemisia Vulgaris*) Oil

Mullein (*Verbascum Thapsus*) Extract

Mushroom (*Corthellus Shiitake*) Extract

Musk Rose (*Rosa Moschata*) Oil

Musk Rose (*Rosa Moschata*) Seed Oil

Myrrh (*Commiphora Myrrha*) Extract

Myrrh (*Commiphora Myrrha*) Oil

Myrrh (*Commiphora Myrrha*) Powder

Myrtle (*Myrtus Communis*) Oil

Neem (*Azadirachta Indica*) Extract

Neem (*Azadirachta Indica*) Leaf Extract

Neem (*Azadirachta Indica*) Seed Oil

Neroli; Bitter Orange (*Citrus Aurantium Amara*) Oil

Nettle (*Urtica Dioica*) Extract

Nettle (*Urtica Dioica*) Oil

Niaouli (*Melaleuca Leucadendron Viridiflora*) Oil

Nori Seaweed (*Fucus Vesiculosis*)

Nori Seaweed (*Fucus Vesiculosis*) Extract

Norway Spruce (*Picea Excelsa*) Extract

Norway Spruce (*Picea Excelsa*) Needle Extract

Norway Spruce (*Picea Excelsa*) Oil

Nutmeg (*Myristica Fragrans*) Extract

Nutmeg (*Myristica Fragrans*) Oil

Oakmoss (*Evernia Prunastri*) Extract

Oat (*Avena Sativa*) Bran

Oat (*Avena Sativa*) Extract

Oat (*Avena Sativa*) Flour

Oat (*Avena Sativa*) Meal

Oat (*Avena Sativa*) Starch

Oatstraw Powder (*Avena Sativa*) Leaf Powder

Olibanum (*Boswellia Carterii*) Extract

Olive (*Olea Europaea*) Oil

Onion (*Allium Cepa*) Extract

Orange (*Citrus Aurantium Dulcis*) Extract

Orange (*Citrus Aurantium Dulcis*) Flower Extract

Orange (*Citrus Aurantium Dulcis*) Flower Oil

Orange (*Citrus Aurantium Dulcis*) Flower Water

Orange (*Citrus Aurantium Dulcis*) Oil

Orange (*Citrus Aurantium Dulcis*) Peel Extract

Orange Oxide (Iron Oxide [and] Glycerin)

Oregano (*Oreganum Vulgare*) Leaf Oil

Orris (*Iris Florentina*) Root Powder

Palm (*Elaeis Guineensis*) Kernel Oil

Palm (*Elaeis Guineensis*) Oil

Palma Christi (*Ricinus Communis*)

Palmarosa (*Cymbopogon Martini*) Oil

Pansy (*Viola Tricolor*) Extract

Papaya (*Carica Papaya*)

Papaya (*Carica Papaya*) Extract

Papaya (*Carica Papaya*) Leaf Extract

Parsley (*Carum Petroselinum*) Extract

Parsley (*Carum Petroselinum*) Seed Oil

Passionflower (*Passiflora Incarnata*) Oil

Patchouli (*Pogostemon Cablin*) Extract

Patchouli (*Pogostemon Cablin*) Oil

Pawpaw (*Asimina Triloba*) Extract

Peach (*Prunus Persica*) Kernel Oil

Peaches N Cream (Mica [and] Titanium Dioxide [and] Glycerin)

Peanut (*Arachis Hypogaea*) Oil

Pecan (*Carya Illinoensis*) Oil

Pelargonium Graveolens Oil (Geranium Oil)

Pellitory (*Parietaria Officinalis*) Extract

Pengawar Djambi (*Cibotium Barometz*) Oil

Pennyroyal (*Mentha Pulegium*) Extract

Pennyroyal (*Mentha Pulegium*) Oil

Pentadesma Butyracea Butter

Pentaerythrityl Tetraoctanoate

Peony (*Paeonia Albiflora*) Extract

Peony (*Paeonia Albiflora*) Root Extract

Peppermint (*Mentha Piperita*) Extract

Peppermint (*Mentha Piperita*) Oil

Peppermint (*Mentha Piperita*) Water

Perfumer's (SD Alcohol 40B) Alcohol

Perilla Ocymoides Extract

Periwinkle (*Vinca Minor*) Extract

Persimmon (*Diospyros Kaki*) Extract

Persimmon (*Diospyros Kaki*) Leaf Extract

Persimmon (*Diospyros Kaki*) Leaf Powder

Peru Balsam (*Myroxylon Balsamum*) Resin

Petitgrain (*Citrus Aurantium*) Oil

Petroleum (*Petrolatum*) Jelly Phenonip (Phenoxyethanol, Methylparaben, Ethylparaben, Butylparaben, Propylparaben, Isobutylparaben)

Pilewort (*Ranunculus Ficaria*) Extract

Pine (*Pinus Haeda*) Bark Extract

Pine (*Pinus Koraiensis*) Extract

Pine (*Pinus Palustris*) Needle Extract

Pine (*Pinus Palustris*) Oil

Pine (*Pinus Palustris*) Tar

Pine (*Pinus Palustris*) Tar Oil

Pine (*Pinus Pinea*) Kernel Oil

Pine (*Pinus Pumilio*) Bark Extract

Pine (*Pinus Pumilio*) Needle Extract

Pine (*Pinus Pumilio*) Oil

Pine (*Pinus Sylvestris*) Bud Extract

Pine (*Pinus Sylvestris*) Cone Extract

Pine (*Pinus Sylvestris*) Cone Oil

Pine (*Pinus Sylvestris*) Needle Extract

Pineapple (*Ananas Sativus*) Extract

Pistachio (*Pistacia Vera*) Nut Oil

Plantain (*Plantago Lanceolata*) Extract

Plantain (*Plantago Major*) Extract

Plantain (*Plantago Ovata*) Extract

Plantain (*Plantago Ovata*) Seed Extract

Plectranthus Barbatus Extract

Plum (*Prunus Domestica*) Extract

Plumeria Alba Extract

Plumeria Rubra Extract

Poke Root (*Phytolacca Decandra*) Extract

Polawax (Emulsifying Wax NF)

Polysorbate 20 NF

Polysorbate 60 NF

Polysorbate 80 NF

Pomegranate (*Punica Granatum*) Extract

Poppy (*Papaver Somniferum*) Seed

Potassium Sorbate

Potato (*Solanum Tuberosum*) Starch

Pretty N Pink (Mica [and] Titanium Dioxide [and] Glycerin)

Prickly Ash (*Zanthoxylum Americanum*) Extract

Prickly Pear (*Opuntia Tuna*) Extract

Propylene Glycol

Pumice

Pumpkin (*Cucurbita Pepo*) Seed Oil

Purple Heath (*Erica Cinerea*) Extract

Quercus Petraea Extract

Quillaja Saponaria Extract

Quince (*Pyrus Cydonia*) Extract

Quince (*Pyrus Cydonia*) Seed

Quinoa (*Chenopodium Quinoa*) Extract

Quinoa (*Chenopodium Quinoa*) Oil

Rapeseed (*Brassica Campestris*) Oil

Raspberry (*Rubus Idaeus*) Seed Oil

Raspberry (*Rubus Suavissimus*) Extract

Raspberry Red (Mica [and] Iron Oxide [and] Titanium Dioxide [and] Glycerin)

Ravensara (*Ravensara Aromatica*) Oil

Red Clay (Montmorillonite)

Red Sandalwood (*Pterocarpus Santalinus*) Extract

Rice (*Oryza Sativa*) Bran Oil

Rice (*Oryza Sativa*) Starch

Rocket (*Eruca Sativa*) Extract

ROE (Rosemary Oleoresin Extract)

Roman Chamomile (*Anthemis Nobilis*) Flower Oil

Rosa Spinosissima Extract

Rose (*Rosa Damascena*) Distillate

Rose (*Rosa Multiflora*) Extract

Rose Absolute (*Rosa Centifolia*) Flower Extract

Rose Geranium (*Pelargonium Graveolens*) Oil

Rosemary (*Rosmarinus Officinalis*) Leaf Extract—ROE

Rosemary (*Rosmarinus Officinalis*) Leaf Powder

Rosemary (*Rosmarinus Officinalis*) Oil

Rosewood (*Aniba Rosaedora*) Extract

Rosewood (*Aniba Rosaedora*) Oil

Rosin

Rowdy Red (Iron Oxide [and] Glycerin)

Safflower (*Carthamus Tinctorius*) Oil

Saffron Crocus (*Crocus Sativus*) Extract

Sage (*Salvia Officinalis*) Extract

Sage (*Salvia Officinalis*) Oil

Sage (*Salvia Officinalis*) Water

Saint John's Wort (INCI of oil used for infusion [and] *Hypericum Perforatum* Flower Extract)

Sal Butter (*Shorea Robusta*) Seed Butter

Salt (all) (Sodium Chloride)

Sandalwood (*Santalum Album*) Oil

Sarsaparilla (*Smilax Aristolochiaefolia*) Extract

Sarsaparilla (*Smilax Utilis*) Extract

Sassafras Officinale Oil

Savory (*Satureia Hortensis*) Extract

Saw Palmetto (*Serenoa Serrulata*) Extract

Schizandra Chinensis Extract

Scotch Pine (*Pinus Sylvestris*) Leaf Oil

Scurvy Grass (*Cochlearia Officinalis*) Extract

Scutellaria Baicalensis Extract

SD Alcohol 40B

Sea Rocket (*Cakile Maritima*) Extract

Seabuckthorn (*Hippophae Rhamnoides*) Oil

Seaweed (*Fucus Vesiculosis*)

Seaweed (*Fucus Vesiculosis*) Extract

Senega (*Polygala Senega*) Extract

Serpentaria (*Aristolochia Clematis*) Extract

Sesame (*Sesamum Indicum*) Oil

Sesame (*Sesamum Indicum*) Seed

Shea (*Butyrospermum Parkii*) Butter

Shepherds Purse (*Capsella Bursa-Pastoris*) Extract

Shield Fern (*Dryopteris Filix-Mas*) Extract

Silk, Hydrolyzed

Silk Amino Acids

Silver Fir (*Abies Pectinata*) Extract

Silver Fir (*Abies Pectinata*) Oil

Sisal (*Agave Rigida*)

Sisal (*Agave Rigida*) Extract

Sisymbrium Irio Oil

Skullcap (*Scutellaria Galericulata*) Extract

Slippery Elm (*Ulmus Fulva*) Bark

Slippery Elm (*Ulmus Fulva*) Extract

Soapberry (*Sapindus Mukurossi*) Extract

Soapberry (*Sapindus Mukurossi*) Peel Extract

Sodium Benzoate

Sodium Lactate

Solanum Lycocarpum Extract

Solomon's Seal (*Polygonatum Multiflorum*) Extract

Solomon's Seal (*Polygonatum Officinale*) Extract

Sophora Japonica Extract

Sorbus (*Pyrus Sorbus*) Extract

Sorrel (*Rumex Acetosella*) Extract

Southernwood (*Artemisia Abrotanum*) Extract

Soybean (*Glycine Soja*) Oil

Spanish Moss (*Tillandsia Usneoides*) Extract

Spanish Pellitory (*Anacyclus Pyrethrum*) Extract

Spanish Rosemary (*Rosmarinus Officinalis*) Leaf Oil

Spearmint (*Mentha Viridis*) Extract

Spearmint (*Mentha Viridis*) Leaf Powder

Spearmint (*Mentha Viridis*) Oil

Spike Lavender (*Lavandula Spica*) Oil

Spinach (*Spinacia Oleracea*) Extract

Spruce (*Tsuga Canadensis*) Leaf Oil

Star of Bethlehem (*Ornithogalum Umbellatum*) Extract

Stearate (Sorbitan Stearate)

Stearic Acid

Stearyl Alcohol

Stevia (*Eupatorium Rebaudianum Bertoni*) Leaf Extract

Stoneroot (*Collinsonia Canadensis*)

Stoneroot (*Collinsonia Canadensis*) Extract

Stramonium (*Datura Stramonium*)

Stramonium (*Datura Stramonium*) Extract

Strawberry (*Fragaria Chiloensis*) Extract

Strawberry (*Fragaria Vesca*)

Strawberry (*Fragaria Vesca*) Extract

Strawberry (*Fragaria Vesca*) Juice

Strawberry (*Fragaria Vesca*) Leaf Extract

Strawberry (*Fragaria Vesca*) Seed

Sugar (Sucrose)

Sugar Cane (*Saccharum Officinarum*) Extract

Sugar Maple (*Acer Saccharinum*) Extract

Sulfated Castor Oil (*Sulfated Ricinus Communis*) Seed Oil—also known as Turkey Red

Sumac (*Rhus Glabra*) Extract

Sunflower (*Helianthus Annuus*) Seed Oil

Sunflower Yellow (Iron Oxide [and] Titanium Dioxide [and] Glycerin)

Sunny Orange (Iron Oxide [and] Titanium Dioxide [and] Glycerin)

Sweet Almond (*Prunus Amygdalus Dulcis*) Oil

Sweet Birch (Methyl Salicylate) Oil

Sweet Cherry (*Prunus Avium*) Pit Oil

Sweet Clover (*Melilotus Officinalis*) Extract

Sweet Fennel (*Foeniculum Vulgare*) Oil

Sweet Grass (*Hierochloe Odorata*) Extract

Sweet Marjoram (*Origanum Majorana*) Extract

Sweet Marjoram (*Origanum Majorana*) Oil

Sweet Orange (*Citrus Aurantium Dulcis*) Oil

Sweet Violet (*Viola Odorata*) Extract

Sweet Violet (*Viola Odorata*) Oil

T-50 (Tocopheryl)

Tagetes (*Tagetes Minuta*) Flower Oil

Talc

Tallow

Tamanu (*Calophyllum Inophyllum*) Oil

Tamarind (*Tamarindus Indica*) Extract

Tamarind (*Tamarindus Indica*) Seed Polysaccharide

Tangerine (*Citrus Tangerina*) Extract

Tansy (*Tanacetum Vulgare*) Extract

Tarragon (*Artemisia Dracunculus*) Extract

TEA (Triethanolamine)

Tea Tree (*Melaleuca Alternifolia*) Oil

Tecoma Curialis Extract

Tecoma Lapacho Extract

Terminalia Catappa Extract

Tetrasodium EDTA

Thaumatococcus Danielli Extract

Thuja Occidentalis Extract

Thuja Occidentalis Oil

Thyme (*Thymus Vulgaris*) Extract

Thyme (*Thymus Vulgaris*) Oil

Tiare (*Gardenia Tahitensis*) Flower

Tiare (*Gardenia Tahitensis*) Flower Extract

Titanium Dioxide

Tomato (*Solanum Lycopersicum*) Juice

Tomato (*Solanum Lycopersicum*) Purée

Tormentil (*Potentilla Erecta*) Extract

Tragacanth (*Astragalus Gummifer*) Extract

Tragacanth (*Astragalus Gummifer*) Gum

Trailing Arbutus (*Epigaea Repens*) Extract

Tuberose (*Polianthes Tuberosa*) Extract

Tunisian Rosemary (*Rosmarinus Officinalis*) Leaf Oil

Turkey Red (*Sulfated Ricinus Communis*) Seed Oil

Turmeric (*Curcuma Longa*) Extract

Turmeric (*Curcuma Longa*) Powder

Turnera Diffusa Extract

Tussilago Vulgaris Extract

Tween 20 (Polysorbate 20)

Tween 60 (Polysorbate 60)

Tween 80 (Polysorbate 80)

Ultramarine Blue Oxide (Iron Oxide)

Ultramarine Pink Oxide (Iron Oxide)

Urtica Urens Extract

Valerian (*Valeriana Officinalis*) Root Oil

Vanilla Planifolia Extract

Vanilla Tahitensis Extract

Vetiver (*Vitiveria Zizanoides*) Oil

Violets Are Blue (Ext. Violet 2 [and] Polyester 3 [and] Titanium Dioxide [and] Glycerin)

Vitamin E (Tocopheryl) Acetate or (Tocopherol) Natural

Walnut (*Juglans Regia*) Extract

Walnut (*Juglans Regia*) Oil

Walnut (*Juglans Regia*) Shell Powder

Water (Aqua)

Water Chestnut (*Eleocharis Dulcis*) Extract

Water Lily (*Nymphaea Alba*) Extract

Water Lily (*Nymphaea Alba*) Root Extract

Water Lily (*Nymphaea Odorata*) Root Extract

Watercress (*Nasturtium Officinale*) Extract

Wheat (*Triticum Vulgare*) Germ Oil

Wheat (*Triticum Vulgare*) Starch

White Camphor (*Cinnamomum Camphora*) Bark Oil

White Ginger (*Hedychium Coronarium*) Extract

White Lily (*Lilium Candidum*) Extract

White Mustard (*Brassica Alba*) Extract

White Nettle (*Lamium Album*) Extract

White Oak (*Quercus Alba*) Bark Extract

White Saponaria (*Gypsophila Paniculata*) Extract

Wild Agrimony (*Potentilla Anserina*) Extract

Wild Cherry (*Prunus Serotina*)

Wild Cherry (*Prunus Serotina*) Bark Extract

Wild Cherry (*Prunus Serotina*) Extract

Wild Indigo (*Baptisia Tinctoria*)

Wild Indigo (*Baptisia Tinctoria*) Extract

Wild Marjoram (*Origanum Vulgare*) Extract

Wild Mint (*Mentha Arvensis*) Extract

Wild Mint (*Mentha Arvensis*) Oil

Wild Mint (*Mentha Arvensis*) Powder

Wild Sarsaparilla (*Aralia Nudicaulis*) Extract

Wild Thyme (*Thymus Serpillum*) Extract

Wild Yam (*Dioscorea Villosa*) Extract

Willow (*Salix Alba*) Bark Extract

Willow (*Salix Alba*) Flower Extract

Willow (*Salix Alba*) Leaf Extract

Willow (*Salix Nigra*) Extract

Wintergreen (*Gaultheria Procumbens*) Extract

Witch Hazel (*Hamamelis Virginiana*) Distillate

Witch Hazel (*Hamamelis Virginiana*) Extract

Woodruff (*Asperula Odorata*) Extract

Xanthan Gum

Ximenia Americana Oil

Yarrow (*Achillea Millefolium*) Extract

Yarrow (*Achillea Millefolium*) Oil

Yerba Santa (*Eriodictyon Crassifolium*) Extract

Ylang-Ylang (*Cananga Odorata*) Oil

Yucca Glauca Extract

Zanthoxylum Piperitum Extract

Zedoary (*Curcuma Zedoaria*) Oil

Zinc Oxide

Zingiber Officinalis

Zizyphus Joaseiro Extract

FDA Labeling Rules

The Food and Drug Administration (FDA) has very strong guidelines when it comes to correctly labeling beauty products. If you're caught without the proper labeling, you will get slapped with a fine.

There is so much controversy on our Yahoo! soap-makers' groups over this issue that we felt the best way to tackle this subject was to give you the links to the FDA sites so you can read them yourselves and make your own interpretations.

The following is just a small sample of the FDA's rules and regulations. Read the rulings carefully, and be sure your labels are in complete compliance.

If you're not in the United States, be sure you find the regulations that apply in your country.

FDA Cosmetic Labeling Manuals and Guides

Following the rules for labeling cosmetics isn't as difficult as you might be thinking right about now. In a nutshell, all the ingredients have to be listed by their INCI names and in order from the most to the least in amount. Most lotions and creams have 50 to 75 percent distilled water, so distilled water would be the very first ingredient listed on the label. Anything under 1 percent does not have to be listed on the label.

The following links give you more information:

"Summary of Regulatory Requirements for Labeling of Cosmetics Marketed in the United States"
www.fda.gov/Cosmetics/CosmeticLabelingLabelClaims/CosmeticLabelingManual/ucm126438.htm

"Labeling Regulations Applicable to Cosmetics"
www.fda.gov/Cosmetics/CosmeticLabelingLabelClaims/CosmeticLabelingManual/ucm126440.htm

"Cosmetic Labeling Guide"
www.fda.gov/Cosmetics/CosmeticLabelingLabelClaims/CosmeticLabelingManual/
ucm126444.htm

"Is It a Cosmetic, a Drug, or Both? (Or Is It Soap?)"
www.fda.gov/Cosmetics/GuidanceComplianceRegulatoryInformation/ucm074201.htm

"How does the law define a cosmetic?"
www.fda.gov/Cosmetics/GuidanceComplianceRegulatoryInformation/ucm074201.htm

"Cosmetics Q&A: 'Personal Care Products'"
www.fda.gov/Cosmetics/ResourcesForYou/Consumers/CosmeticsQA/default.htm

"Are All Personal Care Products Regulated as Cosmetics?"
www.fda.gov/Cosmetics/ResourcesForYou/Consumers/CosmeticsQA/ucm136560.htm

Other Helpful Information

Gale, Marie. *Soap and Cosmetic Labeling: How to Follow the Rules and Regs, Explained in Plain English.* Broadbent, OR: Cinnabar Press, 2007.

Resources

In this appendix, we've assembled a list of some of our favorite venders to help you find the supplies and ingredients you'll need when making your own natural beauty products.

Aloe Vera

Warren Laboratories, LLC
1656 IH 35 South
Abbott, TX 76621
254-580-9990
fax: 254-580-9944
www.warrenlabsaloe.com

Colorants

Apples, Woods and Berries
www.awbsupplies.com

Ellen's Essentials
Houston, TX 77072
www.ellensessentials.com

Select Shades
www.selectshades.com/chart/clear.html

TKB Trading, LLC
1101 9th Avenue
Oakland, CA 94606
510-451-9011
fax: 510-451-4377
tkbtrading@sbcglobal.net
www.tkbtrading.com

Essential Oils

Camden-Grey
3579 NW 82 Avenue
Doral, FL 33122
305-500-9630 or 1-866-503-8615
fax: 305-500-9425
www.camdengrey.com

Stony Mountain Botanicals
www.wildroots.com

Herbs

HerbalCom
3408 Brook Run Drive
Des Moines, IA 50317
1-888-649-3931
fax: 877-818-4115
www.herbalcom.com

Monterey Bay Spice Company
719 Swift Street, Suite 62
Santa Cruz, CA 95060
831-426-2808 or 1-800-500-6148
fax: 831-426-2792
support@herbco.com
www.herbco.com

Oils and Butters

Neem and Karanja Oil and Products
The Ahimsa Alternative, Inc.
Contact: Usha Rao
15 Timberglade Road
Bloomington, MN 55437
952-943-9449 or 1-877-873-6336
fax: 866-211-5460
neemlady@neemresource.com
www.neemresource.com

Oils by Nature, Inc.
30300 Solon Industrial Parkway, Suite E
Solon, OH 44139
440-498-1180
fax: 440-498-0574
info@oilsbynature.com
www.oilsbynature.com

Soaper's Choice
A division of Columbus Foods
Company
Contact: Mike Lawson
30 East Oakton Avenue
Des Plaines, IL 60018
773-265-6500 or 1-800-322-6457
www.soaperschoice.com

Fragrance Oils

Fragrance Oil Finder
www.fragranceoilfinder.com

General Supplies

After the Rayne Supplies
www.atrsupplies.com

Apples, Woods and Berries
903-356-6884
www.awbsupplies.com

Bramble Berry, Inc.
2138 Humboldt Street
Bellingham, WA 98225
(not open to the public)
360-734-8278 or 1-877-627-7883
fax: 360-752-0992
www.brambleberry.com

Elements Bath and Body Supplies
4203 Evergreen Road
Crestwood, KY 40014
502-243-2312
www.elementsbathandbody.com

The Herbarie at Stoney Hill Farm, Inc.
630 Turner Road
Prosperity, SC 29127
803-364-9979 or 1-866-364-9979
fax: 803-364-9974
support@theherbarie.com
www.theherbarie.com

Kangaroo Blue
PO Box 9021
Naperville, IL 60567-9021
630-999-8132
fax: 847-589-1079
www.kangaroblue.com

Lotioncrafter
532 Point Lawrence Road
Olga, WA 98279-8008
sales@lotioncrafter.com
www.lotioncrafter.com

Majestic Mountain Sage
918 West 700 North, Suite 104
Logan, UT 84321
435-766-0863
fax: 435-755-2108
www.thesage.com

Mountain Rose Herbs
PO Box 50220
Eugene, OR 97405
1-800-879-3337 *(outside the USA: 541-741-7307)*
fax: 510-217-4012
info@mountainroseherbs.com
www.mountainroseherbs.com

New Directions Aromatics Inc.
2129 Watercress Place
San Ramon, CA 94583
1-800-246-7117
fax: 1-800-246-8207
www.newdirectionsaromatics.com

Oregon Trail Soap Supplies and More
PO Box 669
Rogue River, OR 97537
541-582-3393
www.oregontrailsoaps.com

The Original Soap Dish
PO Box 263
South Whitney, IN 46787
260-723-4039
www.thesoapdish.com

Taylored Concepts Inc.
12021 Plano Road, Suite #190
Dallas, TX 75243
972-671-5661 or 1-866-322-9944
www.tayloredconcepts.com

Wholesale Supplies Plus, Inc.
10035 Broadview Road
Broadview Heights, OH 44147
440-526-6556 or 1-800-359-0944
fax: 440-526-6597
www.wholesalesuppliesplus.com

Labels and Packaging Supplies

BayouSome.com
385 Farmer Court, Suite A
Lawrenceville, GA 30046
service@bayousome.com
www.bayousome.com

Elements Bath and Body Supplies
4203 Evergreen Road
Crestwood, KY 40014
502-243-2312
www.elementsbathandbody.com

Online Labels, Inc.
925 Florida Central Parkway
Longwood, FL 32750
407-949-6499 or 1-888-575-2235
fax: 1-866-406-7341
www.onlinelabels.com

The Shrink Wrap Store
www.shrinkwrapstore.com

Wholesale Supplies Plus, Inc.
www.wholesalesuppliesplus.com

Preservatives

Do you need to use a preservative? The short answer is "yes." Even if you're not planning on selling your beauty products and intend them only for yourself and family, know this: bacteria can grow in a lotion or cream without a single indicator or odor. You won't even know if a product is tainted until it's too late. Your eyes, for example, can become infected with the smallest amount of cream that has bacteria growing in it.

Always preserve your products, and if you're going to sell them, have them tested.

Choosing Your Preservative

You'll find many preservatives available, and it can boggle your mind trying to decide which is best for what you want to preserve. I wish I could give you just one preservative that would work in all cases. But unfortunately, that's not possible.

There are several factors to consider when choosing a preservative. One is the pH of the product you need to preserve. Some of the preservatives work in low pH, while some work in all ranges of pH. So take note of your product's pH levels when you're deciding which preservative you should use.

You can use preservatives high in parabens and preserve a product until the end of time. But I don't use parabens or formaldehyde in anything I make. There are too many links to damaged breast tissues from products that contain parabens. There are many who say there's not enough proof that they're dangerous, but still, I avoid them. Read what these preservatives are made of, and take the time to research what these chemicals are before you make your decisions.

The following sections are broken down into which emulsion needs which preservative. Each preservative includes its INCI name, the amount you'll use of the preservative, with what pH range it works or doesn't work, what temperature your emulsion should be to mix in the preservative, and if it is a *total preservative*.

Unless otherwise noted, all these preservatives are produced by ISP Corporation.

Anhydrous Preservatives

These are for formulations that don't include water (you'll need a preservative specially designed for this). Formulations such as simple body butters whipped with only the butters and an oil require this type of preservative.

LiquaPar MEP   INCI: Phenoxyethanol (and) Methylparaben (and) Ethylparaben (and) Propylparaben. Effective against gram-positive and gram-negative bacteria, yeast, and mold. Use .5 to 1 percent. pH levels: 3 to 7.5. Don't use in nonionic surfactants and emulsifiers. Add at the coolest temperature possible. When making a formulation at cold or room temperature, add early in the process.

LiquaPar Oil   INCI: Isopropylparaben (and) Isobutylparaben (and) Butylparaben. Effective against gram-positive bacteria, yeast, and mold, but not against gram-negative bacteria. Use .4 to .8 percent. Can be added before or after emulsification in formulations that have a pH range of 3 to 7.5.

LiquaPar Optima   INCI: Phenoxyethanol (and) Methylparaben (and) Isopropylparaben (and) Isobutylparaben (and) Butylparaben. This total preservative works against gram-positive and gram-negative bacteria, yeast, and mold. Use .5 to 1 percent, in a formulation that has a pH range of 3 to 7.5. Use the coolest temperature possible when adding this preservative. For cold or room temperature–mixed formulas, add early in the process.

LiquaPar PE   INCI: Phenoxyethanol (and) Isopropylparaben (and) Isobutylparaben (and) Butylparaben. This total preservative is effective against gram-positive and gram-negative bacteria, yeast, and mold, providing broad-spectrum protection. Use .5 to 1 percent. Works in formulas within a pH range of 3 to 7.5. Use the coolest temperature possible when adding this preservative. If you have a more complex formula, use 1 percent LiquaPar PE and also add .2 percent ethylenediaminetetraacetic acid salt (EDTA).

LiquaPar PN   INCI: Phenoxyethanol (and) Methylparaben (and) Ethylparaben (and) Propylparaben (and) Butylparaben. Use .5 to 1 percent, in a pH range of 3 to 7.5. For more complex formulas, use 1 percent LiquaPar PN with .2 percent ethylenedi-aminetetraacetic acid salt (EDTA). Use the coolest possible temperature when adding this preservative.

Water-Soluble Preservatives

This group of preservatives dissolves in products with water. Think shower gels, shampoo gel, and laundry soap. Also good in products that do not use an emulsifier.

Germall II   INCI: Diazolidinyl Urea (a formaldehyde-releasing preservative). This white powder provides a wide range of antibacterial protection from gram-positive and gram-negative organisms. To have across-the-board protection from yeast and mold, you need to add methylparaben and propylparaben. Use .1 to .3 percent, in a pH range from 3 to 9.

Germall 115   INCI: Imidazolidinyl Urea (a formaldehyde-releasing preservative). This is effective against gram-positive and gram-negative bacteria, but does not protect against yeast and mold contamination. Use up to .6 percent of the total weight in a wide pH range, from 3 to 9.

Germall Plus   INCI: Diazolidinyl Urea (and) Iodopropynyl Butylcarbamate. This broad-spectrum total preservative protects against gram-positive and gram-negative bacteria, plus yeast and mold, and is in powder form. Germall Plus is 99 percent diazolidinyl urea (formaldehyde), 1 percent iodopropynyl butylcarbamate. Use .05 to .2 percent in a wide pH of 3 to 9. It can be used in products with proteins and cationic, anionic, or nonionic surfactants and emulsifiers.

Emulsion Preservatives

These are preservatives for products in which you've used an emulsifier—think lotions and creams.

Germaben II   INCI: Propylene Glycol (and) Diazolidinyl Urea (and) Methylparaben (and) Propylparaben. This preservative contains formaldehyde (diazolidinyl urea) with parabens. It is effective against gram-positive and gram-negative bacteria, yeast, and mold, and can be used in shampoos, hair conditioners, and emulsion products. Use .5 to 1 percent; pH 3 to 7.5.

Germaben II-E   INCI: Propylene Glycol (and) Diazolidinyl Urea (and) Methylparaben (and) Propylparaben. It is a broad-spectrum, total preservative. Use .5 to 1 percent; pH range 3 to 7.5. Designed for emulsion systems with oil phases greater than 25 percent. Mix into your formula at the coolest temperature possible.

Optiphen   INCI: Phenoxyethanol (and) Caprylyl Glycol. Optiphen is a paraben-free and formaldehyde-free liquid preservative. Use .75 to 1.5 percent; no pH restrictions. Mix into your formula at the coolest temperature possible.

Optiphen ND   INCI: Phenoxyethanol (and) Benzoic Acid (and) Dehydroacetic Acid. Optiphen ND is an across-the-board, liquid total preservative that does not contain formaldehyde or formaldehyde releasers, and is paraben-free. It is effective against gram-positive and gram-negative bacteria, yeast, and mold. Use .2 to 1.2 percent; the pH of finished formulations should be 6 or below. Mix into your formula at the coolest temperature possible.

Optiphen Plus   INCI: Phenoxyethanol (and) Caprylyl Glycol (and) Sorbic Acid. This is a broad-spectrum, total preservative. Use .75 to 1.5 percent. It performs best in formulations below a pH of 6, but depending on the formula, it has also proven effective when used in formulas with pH levels above 6. Add to formulas at cool temperatures.

Natural Preservatives

Several different companies are working on natural preservatives that can be used in cosmetics; one company is even using oregano as the base for their preservative. Ciba Specialty Chemicals is one such company. Go to www.naturalingredient.org/Articles/Tinosan_Micro_info.pdf to see what they've been up to.

This company produces Tinosan SDC, which is a new antimicrobial preservative made from silver and citric acid. It's a broad-spectrum antimicrobial that's effective against bacteria and microorganisms. Tinosan SDC is water-soluble and easy to use in the water phase of gels, surfactants, and emulsions made at room temperature. When making products that have to be heated, such as melting waxes and butters, add Tinosan at the coolest possible temperature. The use rate is .03 to .1 percent.

What Preservative to Use When?

For your convenience, we have this quick-glance guide to help you:

For wet wipes, use Liquid Germall Plus, Suttocide A, Optiphen ND, or Optiphen Plus.

For clear gels, use Germall Plus, Liquid Germall Plus, or Suttocide A.

For low-pH products, use Germall Plus, Liquid Germall Plus, Optiphen ND, or Optiphen Plus.

LiquaGard works synergistically with a number of the preservatives to boost antifungal properties. Used with the following ISP preservatives, you can achieve broad-spectrum preservation protection for your final formula:

Germall 115

Germall II

Optiphen

Optiphen ND

Optiphen Plus

Suttocide A

Index